Forced Migration in the History of 20th Century Neuroscience and Psychiatry

The forced migration of neuroscientists, both during and after the Second World War, is of growing interest to international scholars. Of particular interest is how the long-term migration of scientists and physicians has affected both the academic migrants and their receiving environments. As well as the clash between two different traditions and systems, this migration forced scientists and physicians to confront foreign institutional, political, and cultural frameworks when trying to establish their own ways of knowledge generation, systems of logic, and cultural mentalities.

The twentieth century has been called the century of war and forced-migration, since it witnessed two devastating world wars, prompting a massive exodus that included many neuroscientists and psychiatrists. Fascism in Italy and Spain beginning in the 1920s, Nazism in Germany and Austria between the 1930s and 1940s, and the impact of the Soviet occupation of Eastern Europe all forced more than two thousand researchers with prior education in neurology, psychiatry, and the basic brain research disciplines to leave their scientific and academic home institutions. This edited volume, comprising of eight chapters written by international specialists, reflects on the complex dimensions of intellectual migration in the neurosciences and illustrates them by using relevant case studies, biographies, and historical surveys.

This book was originally published as a special issue of the *Journal of the History of the Neurosciences*.

Frank W. Stahnisch is AMF/Hannah Professor in the History of Medicine and Health Care in the Departments of History and Community Health Sciences at the University of Calgary, Canada.

Gül A. Russell is Professor of History of Medicine in the Department of Humanities in Medicine at Texas A&M University, USA.

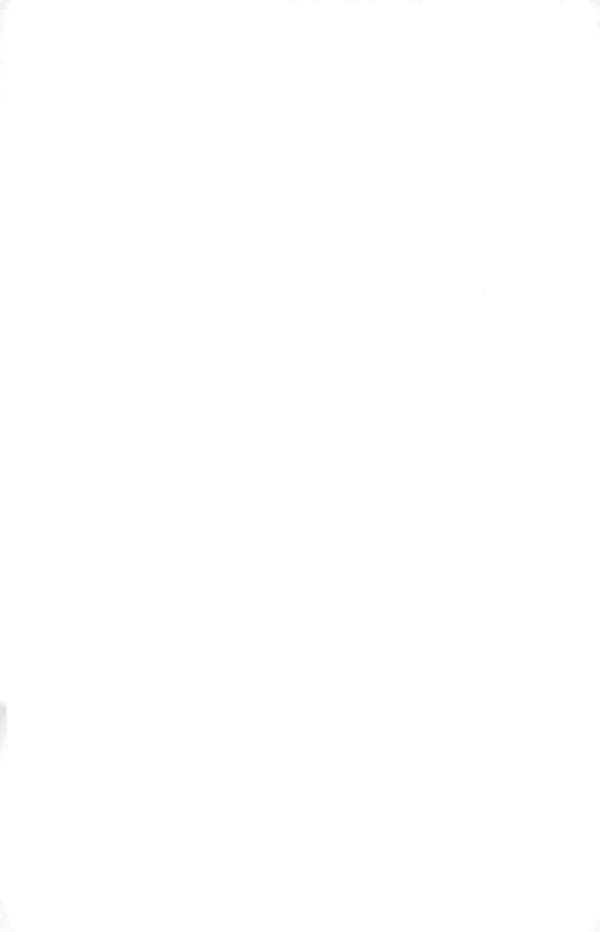

Forced Migration in the History of 20th Century Neuroscience and Psychiatry

New Perspectives

Edited by
Frank W. Stahnisch and Gül A. Russell

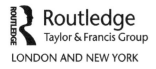

Routledge
Taylor & Francis Group

LONDON AND NEW YORK

First published 2018 by Routledge

2 Park Square, Milton Park, Abingdon, Oxfordshire OX14 4RN
52 Vanderbilt Avenue, New York, NY 10017

Routledge is an imprint of the Taylor & Francis Group, an informa business

First issued in paperback 2019

British Library Cataloguing in Publication Data
A catalogue record for this book is available from the British Library

ISBN 13: 978-1-138-73305-3 (hbk)
ISBN 13: 978-0-367-26474-1 (pbk)

Typeset in Minion Pro
by RefineCatch Limited, Bungay, Suffolk

Publisher's Note
The publisher accepts responsibility for any inconsistencies that may have
arisen during the conversion of this book from journal articles to book chapters,
namely the possible inclusion of journal terminology.

Disclaimer
Every effort has been made to contact copyright holders for their permission to
reprint material in this book. The publishers would be grateful to hear from any
copyright holder who is not here acknowledged and will undertake to rectify
any errors or omissions in future editions of this book.

Contents

Citation Information

The chapters in this book were originally published in the *Journal of the History of the Neurosciences*, volume 25, issue 3 (2016). When citing this material, please use the original page numbering for each article, as follows:

Introduction
New perspectives on forced migration in the history of twentieth-century neuroscience
Frank W. Stahnisch and Gül A. Russell
Journal of the History of the Neurosciences, volume 25, issue 3 (2016), pp. 219–226

Chapter 1
"History had taken such a large piece out of my life" — Neuroscientist refugees from Hamburg during National Socialism
Lawrence A. Zeidman, Anna von Villiez, Jan-Patrick Stellmann, and Hendrik van den Bussche
Journal of the History of the Neurosciences, volume 25, issue 3 (2016), pp. 275–298

Chapter 2
Between resentment and aid: German and Austrian psychiatrist and neurologist refugees in Great Britain since 1933
Aleksandra Loewenau
Journal of the History of the Neurosciences, volume 25, issue 3 (2016), pp. 348–362

Chapter 3
Emigrated neuroscientists from Berlin to North America
Bernd Holdorff
Journal of the History of the Neurosciences, volume 25, issue 3 (2016), pp. 227–252

Chapter 4
Learning soft skills the hard way: Historiographical considerations on the cultural adjustment process of German-speaking émigré neuroscientists in Canada, 1933 to 1963
Frank W. Stahnisch
Journal of the History of the Neurosciences, volume 25, issue 3 (2016), pp. 299–319

Chapter 5

A variation on forced migration: Wilhelm Peters (Prussia via Britain to Turkey) and Muzafer Sherif (Turkey to the United States)
Gül A. Russell
Journal of the History of the Neurosciences, volume 25, issue 3 (2016), pp. 320–347

Chapter 6

Eugenics ideals, racial hygiene, and the emigration process of German-American neurogeneticist Franz Josef Kallmann (1897–1965)
Stephen Pow and Frank W. Stahnisch
Journal of the History of the Neurosciences, volume 25, issue 3 (2016), pp. 253–274

Chapter 7

Émigré scientists and the global turn in the history of science: A commentary on the special issue "New Perspectives on Forced Migration in the History of Twentieth-Century Neuroscience"
Delia Gavrus
Journal of the History of the Neurosciences, volume 25, issue 3 (2016), pp. 363–368

For any permission-related enquiries please visit:
http://www.tandfonline.com/page/help/permissions

Notes on Contributors

Delia Gavrus is Associate Professor and Chancellor's Research Chair at the Department of History, University of Winnipeg, Canada.

Bernd Holdorff is Director Emeritus of the Department of Neurology, Schlosspark-Klinik Berlin, Germany.

Aleksandra Loewenau is a Postdoctoral Fellow at the Department of Community Health Sciences and the Calgary Institute for the Humanities, University of Calgary, Canada.

Stephen Pow is based at the Doctoral School of History, Central European University, Budapest, Hungary.

Gül A. Russell is Professor of History of Medicine in the Department of Humanities in Medicine at Texas A&M University, Health Science Center, College of Medicine, Texas, USA.

Frank W. Stahnisch is AMF/Hannah Professor in the History of Medicine and Health Care in the Departments of History and Community Health Sciences at the University of Calgary, Canada.

Jan-Patrick Stellmann is a Clinical Scientist at the Institute of Neuroimmunology and Multiple Sclerosis and Department of Neurology, University Medical Center Hamburg-Eppendorf, Germany.

Hendrik van den Bussche is Associate Professor at the Institute of Neuroimmunology and Multiple Sclerosis and Department of Neurology, University Medical Center Hamburg-Eppendorf, Germany.

Anna von Villiez is a Research Associate at the Department of History, University of Hamburg, Germany.

Lawrence A. Zeidman is Associate Professor at the Department of Neurology and Rehabilitation, University of Illinois at Chicago College of Medicine, USA.

Preface

Gül A. Russell and Frank W. Stahnisch

The transmigration of scholars and scientists, whether forced or voluntary has been a continuous phenomenon, but an under-researched topic in the longer history of science, medicine, and technology (e.g. Ash & Soellner, 1996). On occasion dramatic cases have drawn scholarly attention, such as Réné Descartes' (1596–1650) escape to the Netherlands in the theologically charged context of science in the seventeenth century (Schuurman, 2004, pp. 56–69). Following the trial of Galileo Galilei (1564–1642) by the ecclesiastical Inquisition, scientists in the Catholic countries were silenced by fear (Langford, 1971, pp. 1–22). It was, however, only during the twentieth century that we have an unprecedented example of both: "forced migration *en masse*" with the Nazi and Fascist expulsion of German-speaking academics in the 1930s and 1940s; and "voluntary" migration—on a quantitatively smaller scale—from England with the increasing hostility to biomedical sciences under the influence of the anti-vivisection movement in the 1980s (e.g. Guither, 1998, pp. 181–200). The concept of "brain drain-brain gain" introduced to describe these historical processes (Medawar & Pyke, 2001), though widely accepted, represents rather the tip of an iceberg that disguises layers of unexplored and at times unexpected complexity (Stahnisch, 2010).

This book provides a critical review and analysis of the multifaceted processes of transmigration, focusing largely on disciplines that relate to the neurosciences.

The in-depth case studies open up a new window into the subject, beyond the reductionist "brain drain-brain gain" equation that has rather acquired the status of a slogan than a serious analytical instrument. The chapters compiled in this volume reveal what it means to be uprooted from a familiar environment, whether personal, social, cultural, linguistic, or professional; the effect of transmigration on the experiences of individuals, the mixed responses of the host societies, their institutions, as well as the particular disciplines of science itself. The individual contributors to the book pose questions that challenge the very nature of objectivity in scholarship, which is based on such a facile concept as "drain" and "gain."

These studies bring out the role of organizations, institutions, and occasionally governments, where the selection process was determined by self-interest and specific "need"; or of the network of scientists themselves, where the concern was with saving the future of science, rather than assisting individual scientists. They identify the problems that the émigrés faced. These were at times insurmountable, at times with tragic consequences—in entering, staying, or getting a position, any position at all, whether or not incommensurate with their previous professional status, or level of expertise.

They analyze the influential factors in hiring practices, not only the economic ones during the aftermath of the Great Depression, for example, but the deeply rooted ethnic prejudices or gender preferences and discriminations (Pearle, 1981). The chapters assembled in this volume were originally published with an introductory overview and commentary, as six articles in the special issue of the *Journal of the History of the Neurosciences*, volume 25:3 (July–September) edited by Frank W. Stahnisch and Guel A. Russell. They constitute only part of the editor-authors' broader concern to explore the twentieth-century phenomena of scientific and medical transmigration in a comprehensive multinational research undertaking.

The editors believe that despite the shifting contexts and locales, there are continuous threads, both culture-specific as well as across geographical boundaries and periods. These are of fundamental importance. They may deepen our understanding of the processes and mechanisms that underlie the varieties of on-going phenomena in our times. They caution us, in the words of the Spanish-American philosopher and poet George Santayana (1863–1952)—that "*Those who do not remember the past are condemned to repeat it*" (Santayana, 1905, p. 284).

The book was conceptualized in July 2013. An interdisciplinary group of scholars from six countries and three continents met during the International Congress of History of Science and Technology (ICHST) at the University of Manchester in the United Kingdom (Stahnisch & Russell, 2013). Under the title of "Knowledge between Transmission and Local Cultural Boundaries: Migrating Scientists and Physicians in the Twentieth Century," they set out to examine issues regarding the forced migration of researchers and scholars under extreme political pressures (e.g. Hobsbawm, 1994). There were two major examples: the German-speaking psychiatrists and neuroscientists during the period of Nazism and Fascism in Europe, who sought refuge in Great Britain and North America, or found one in Turkey through a formal Government invitation; and the Russian natural scientists and physicists, who fled to the United States, Canada, and Latin America, during the Stalin era in the Soviet Union (Marks, Weindling & Wintour, 2011). The individual chapters in the current volume thus bring together the results of several presentations from the conference with additional solicited contributions from both editors that provide new perspectives on the forced migration of particularly German-speaking neurologists, psychiatrists, and psychologists during the first half of the twentieth century.

That this book could eventually come to fruition was due to several institutions and individuals. The editors gratefully acknowledge their role. First of all, the International Congress of History of Science and Technology where Jeff A. Hughes and James Sumner, as the chairs of the local organizing committee, positively reviewed and generously accepted the original scholarly panel at the University of Manchester in 2013. Then, the *Journal of the History of the Neurosciences* where its editors Stanley Finger, Peter J. Koehler, and Marc Macmillan at the time allowed the previous publication of a themed issue entitled "New Perspectives on Forced-Migration in Neuroscience during the Twentieth Century." They immediately recognized an under-studied area of research in scientific transmigration and the need for more analytical case studies, to unravel the underlying complex adaptation processes with individual émigré neurologists, psychiatrists, and psychologists in their new host countries. Previously, the journal had published several articles on a number of influential cases that helped to set the stage for further explorations of forced migration in the history of the neurosciences (e.g. Zeidman & Mohan, 2014; Holdorff, 2002). In this book, the general questions previously raised in other investigations, are also taken up, but reconsidered from their respective social historical, network-analytical, and cultural perspectives.

We are grateful to Dr. Anna Perlina from the Max Planck Institute for the History of Science in Berlin, Germany, who has helped to initiate the project, and seconded the initial planning of the scholarly panel in Manchester in 2013. We would further like to thank Nicholas Barclay of Routledge in London, England, for the review of the manuscript, and his ensuing inclusion of our volume in the history series of this central academic publishing house. The Canadian Institutes for Health Research (CIHR), and its Ethics Office partially supported the research for several of the articles, as well as the organization of the scholarly panel at the International Congress of History of Science and Technology through an Open Operating Grant, entitled "The Cultural Context of Modern Neuroscientific Research: Exploring the Impact of Institutional Research Settings and Professional Migration Patterns" (EOG No. 123690).

Furthermore, Frank W. Stahnisch wishes to thank the University Research Grant Committee of the University of Calgary for the award of a Social Sciences and Humanities Research Council (SSHRC) enhancement grant ("German-Speaking Émigrés-Neuroscientists in Canada and the United States, 1930s to 1970s"). This grant has supported ongoing research into the conditions and the processes of the adaptation and acculturation of émigré neurologists and psychiatrists in Canada and the United States. The Calgary Institute for the Humanities (CIH), under the direction of Dr. Jim Ellis, has also supported a working group on "The Forced-Migration of German-Speaking Neuroscientists and Biomedical Researchers, 1933–1989," co-led by university historian Dr. Paul Stortz, that will help foster national and international collaborations on issues of the forced migration in science, medicine, and technology in the near future. Furthermore, Guel A. Russell wishes to acknowledge support received from Texas A&M University Health Science Center College of Medicine, in particular, Ruth L. Bush, JD, MPH, Vice Dean for Academic Affairs, contributing to the original organization of another scholarly panel at Wadham College, Oxford, and the initial stages of her research on émigré neuropathologists and psychologists in Turkey and the United States.

Finally, we thank all the external reviewers of the individual chapters of the volume for their helpful criticisms, valuable comments, and expedient support for the improvement and finalizing process of the chapters. The editorial assistance of Ms. Aoife Buckley at Taylor & Francis in Philadelphia, Pennsylvania, was invaluable in bringing this project together. Mrs Erna Kurbegović and Dr. Brennan Smith at the University of Calgary, Alberta, further assisted with the editing and language revisions of the international chapters, along with the preformatting of the manuscripts.

References

Ash M, Soellner A, eds. (1996): *Forced Migration and Scientific Change: Émigré German–Speaking Scientists after 1933.* Cambridge, Cambridge University Press.

Guither HD (1998): *Animal Rights: History and Scope of a Radical Social Movement.* Carbondale and Edwardsville, University of Illinois Press.

Hobsbawm E (1994): *The Age of Extremes: The Short Twentieth Century, 1914–1991.* London, Random House.

Holdorff B (2002): Friedrich Heinrich Lewy (1885–1950) and His Work. *Journal of the History of the Neurosciences* 11: 19–28.

Langford JJ (1971): *Galileo, Science and the Church.* Ann Arbor, The University of Michigan.

Marks S, Weindling P, Wintour L, eds. (2011): *In Defence of Learning – The Plight, Persecution, and Placement of Academic Refugees, 1933–1980s.* Oxford, Oxford University Press.

Medawar J, Pyke D (2001): *Hitler's Gift. The True Story of the Scientists Expelled by the Nazi Regime.* New York: Arkade Publishing.

Pearle KM (1981): *Preventive Medicine: The Refugee Physicians and the New York Medical Community 1933–1945* (Working Papers on Blocked Alternatives in the Health Policy System). Bremen, n. loc., 1981.

Santayana G (1905): *The Life of Reason: Reason in Common Sense.* London, Scribner's, 1905.

Schuurman P (2004): *Ideas, Mental Faculties, and Method: The Logic of Ideas of Descartes and Locke and its Reception in the Dutch Republic, 1630–1750.* Leiden, Boston, Brill.

Stahnisch FW, Russell GA (2013): Knowledge between Transmission and Local Cultural Boundaries: Migrating Scientists and Physicians in the Twentieth Century. In: International Congress of History of Science and Technology, ed., *24th ICHST Congress in Manchester.* Manchester: University of Manchester (http://www. ichstm2013.com/programme/guide/s/S065.html), accessed October 1, 2016.

Stahnisch FW (2010): German-Speaking Émigré-Neuroscientists in North America after 1933: Critical Reflections on Emigration-Induced Scientific Change. *Oesterreichische Zeitschrift fuer Geschichtswissenschaften (Vienna)* 21: 36–68.

Zeidman LA, Mohan L (2014): Adolf Wallenberg: Giant in Neurology and Refugee from Nazi Europe. *Journal of the History of the Neurosciences* 23: 31–44.

Forced Migration in the History of 20th-Century Neuroscience and Psychiatry

Frank W. Stahnisch and Gül A. Russell

ABSTRACT

This special issue of the *Journal of the History of the Neurosciences*, comprised of six articles and one commentary, reflects on the multi-fold dimensions of intellectual migration in the neurosciences and illustrates them by relevant case studies, biographies, and surveys from twentieth-century history of science and medicine perspectives. The special issue as a whole strives to emphasize the impact of forced migration in the neurosciences and psychiatry from an interdisciplinary perspective by, first, describing the general research topic, second, by showing how new models can be applied to the historiography and social studies of twentieth-century neuroscience, and, third, by providing a deeper understanding of the impact of European émigré researchers on emerging allied fields, such as neurogenetics, biological psychiatry, psychosomatics, and public mental health, etc. as resulting from this process at large.

The forced migration of hundreds of neuroscientists and thousands of researchers and professors from the Fascist and Nazi-occupied European countries in the first half of the twentieth century still poses a major conundrum for the history of medicine and science today (Ash & Soellner, 1996). Often, the so-called "Brain Gain Thesis" is invoked as an unquestioned given in studies on the forced migration of physicians and medical researchers following the Nazis' rise to power in Germany after 1933. Research literature on the receiving countries has primarily tended to take the intellectual, academic, and institutional dimensions of the forced migration wave into account (Medawar & Pyke, 2001), while the individual fate and adaptation problems of many émigré neurologists and psychiatrists are still fairly underinvestigated. This special issue of the *Journal of the History of the Neurosciences* looks at the fate of a group of émigré physicians and researchers who could be classified as "neuroscientists" widely and who immigrated to the United States, Canada, Britain, and Turkey (Schwartz, 1995) either transitionally or permanently. The thesis put forward here is that the process of forced migration most often constituted an end or at least a drastic change to the career patterns of this group of medical professionals (see also Stahnisch, 2010). Based on historical evidence, the "Brain Gain Thesis" needs to be significantly readjusted as a methodological tool in the field of immigration studies in medicine.

Persecution, emigration, and readaptation of German-speaking Jewish and oppositional neuroscientists and psychiatrists

The forced migration of Jewish and political oppositional physicians and scientists in Germany, as well as later also in Austria and many of the occupied European countries, was primarily brought about by the inauguration of the Nazi Law on the Re-Establishment of the Professional Civil Service (*Gesetz zur Wiederherstellung des Berufsbeamtentums*) from April 7, 1933 (Bleker, 1989). During the same year, when the first refugees reached their new host countries, various scientific and social assistance groups had already been founded, of which the Society for the Protection of Science and Learning (formerly known as the British Assistance Council, which Sir William Henry Beveridge [1879–1963] had initiated in 1933) deserves particular mentioning (Zimmerman, 2006). Yet, unfortunately, in 1933 when the Nazi Party came to power, professional associations such as the "American Medical Association" (AMA), the most influential pressure group for the protection of medical interests in the United States, became themselves engaged in campaigns to constrain the relicensing process for foreign-educated physicians (Pearle, 1981).

This themed issue investigates some important negotiation processes and cultural influences on modern neuroscience with a focus on institutional, organizational, and researcher migration issues. The articles assembled here follow integrated prosopographical, institutional, and network historiographical approaches, while investigating the biographical, conceptual, and organizational information on émigré neuroscientists (cf. Zeidman & Kondziella, 2012), who were ousted from their home countries in the 1930s and 1940s. They came to various new scientific landscapes, primarily in North America, the United Kingdom, Israel (Palestine), and Turkey, which adds a distinctly global perspective to the forced migration movement during the first half of the twentieth century (Strauss & Roeder, 1983). The articles compiled in this special issue further analyze the role of international networks that facilitated the forced migration of the special group of approximately 600 neurologists, psychiatrists, and other medical researchers and clinicians, as well as the subgroup of these refugees that was integrated into North American neuroscience centers, the reciprocal changes of these research settings, and the ways they were locally modified (Niederland, 1988). By applying a cultural view to neuroscience history, the current contributions give new insights into the nature of progressive and regressive factors of individual forms of research organization, the development of institutional models, and their impact on modern neuroscience as a whole. They thereby contribute to the advancement of knowledge in medicine and provide historical information for use among respective stakeholders, such as researchers, administrators, and organizational leaders, about the development and state of the international neurosciences (Magoun, 2002). The underlying topics investigate some major institutional settings and patterns of migration and adaptation in North American neuroscience between the 1930s (when Fascism and Nazism had been at their high point of power in Europe) and the 1950s (when most of the émigré neuroscientists and psychiatrists had actively resettled and reintegrated in the scientific and medical research landscapes of their new home countries), in order to determine its receptiveness to external impulses and its permeability for foreign researchers and physicians.

The exodus of medical doctors and brain researchers as a result of the "de-judification" of German-speaking neuroscience

Nazi ideology, as exemplified in the "Law on the Re-Establishment of the Professional Civil Service" (Longerich, 2010, p. 38) regarded it as unacceptable, and even dangerous, if Arians were taught by Jews, and as a result many university professors, teachers, and doctors of the public health service lost their positions in the German civil service system. Even honorary officials of scientific boards and academic committees were released from their duties (Holdorff & Winau, 2001). Hence, this law cut deeply into the developed culture of science and medicine during the Weimar Republic, now in a cultural and political climate, where the Nazi legal programs and actions became paralleled through the rising dominance of racial hygiene, eugenics, and later even patient euthanasia in psychiatry and neurology (Weindling, 1989). What is further crucial with respect to the emergence—and in this instance largely the destruction—of the new research field of the neurosciences was the active persecution and expulsion of what the Nazis saw as a "Jewish form of medicine and health care" in Germany. This was particularly exemplified by the previous psychoanalytic tradition in psychiatry, socialist public health programs, as well as the emergence of medical sexology (*Sexualwissenschaft*) (Herrn, 2010). The normative context of medicine and psychiatry in the "Third Reich" was such that medical scientists stepped out of their normal doctor–patient relationships and also left deeply engrained professional behavior of mutual respect, while pursuing lines of open antagonism towards their Jewish colleagues and the doctors who openly resented the increasing radicalism and inhuman shape of the medical system.

These changes in the political and organizational structure of the German-speaking medical system became particularly visible in the process of expulsion and later murder of Jewish and non-conformist doctors (Kater, 1989). However, research literature has been primarily concerned with the biographical developments along with the criminal activities of contemporary doctors, while the particular cultural and social context of the Nazi period has been only marginally discussed. It is these developments following 1933, however, that are quite important for the narrative of this special issue including, for example, the loss of medical licenses to practice for individual doctors and clinical researchers, restraints for Jewish neurologists and psychiatrists to exercise their professional and academic rights, as well as the restrictions of medical care applications to Jewish patients only. At the same time, mental asylums, social care facilities, and health education institutions were shut down—representing important preludes to what extended into the greatest exodus of scientists and doctors in European history (Medawar & Pyke, 2001, pp. 231–240).

While the primary focus is laid here on émigré neuroscientists, it needs to be emphasized that not all clinical neurologists, psychiatrists, and laboratory researchers who left Germany and Austria after 1933 were of Jewish descent. Although the numerical data are vacillating on this point, between 10 and 20% of the science émigrés decided to leave Europe for other reasons—out of fear that their relatives could be imprisoned, due to their former political opposition (as socialists, communists, or pacifists), or merely because they had been abroad on research fellowships and decided that things could only get worse for them if they returned to Germany or Austria (Niederland, 1988, pp. 285–300). This is, for example, the case for Berlin biophysicist Max Delbrueck (1906–1981) (who also did important neuro-membrane research), who later became a professor at California Institute of Technology in Pasadena, or Hungarian-born, Viennese-trained Stephen W. Kuffler (1913–1980). Kuffler worked on single nerve-muscle preparation and joined Johns Hopkins University in Baltimore, Maryland, after an extensive period in John Eccles' (1903–1997) laboratory at the University of Otago in New Zealand, where he investigated the neurophysiology of nerve dendrites. Also in this category is the clinical psychiatrist and geriatric physician Erich Lindemann (1900–1974), who arrived in the United States in 1927 and through other appointments later became the chairman of psychiatry at the Massachusetts General Hospital in Boston, Massachusetts, in the United States.

Taking a brief look at the general numbers of the émigré neuroscientists reveals that approximately 2,000 scientists and university professors were expelled from Germany before 1938 (Ash & Soellner, 1996, pp. 23–47). Amongst them were nearly 600 researchers, according to a 1988 survey from the Leo Baeck Institute for the history and culture of German-speaking Jewry, with half of these researchers being fully trained neurologists and psychiatrists (Krohn et al., 1989, pp. 904–1048). This sample represents a highly significant group with respect to Germany as well as in comparison to the new host countries. The registers of the Royal College of Physicians, for example, show the presence of around 200 psychiatrists and several dozen neurologists in the United Kingdom in 1940 and the files of the American Academy of Neurology (AAN) list approximately 500 individuals with specialty training in 1948 (AAN, 1948–1953) after the end of the Second World War. The historical problem of emigration-induced change has been researched from multiple perspectives including the fields of the humanities and social sciences. Not only did they draw on individual biographies and collective biographies but they also measured the "hard impact parameters" like bibliometric methods, memberships in academic associations, and statistics on the leading positions in scholarly societies (Juette, 1990, pp. 17–122).

This sample, therefore, represents a fairly significant group of refugee academics. That this massive loss of researchers had had a disastrous effect on basic and clinical neuroscience in Germany and Austria is self-explanatory, while some authors have interpreted these occurrences simply as a matter of "brain loss" for German-speaking science and in terms of the brain gain thesis for the rest of the world (Medawar & Pyke, 2001, pp. 231–240). Although this view might not be entirely wrong, it fails to provide us with the full complexity of the processes involved, and, too often, individual gains came at a significant loss—for clinical medicine, biomedical research, and psychiatric practice, as well as many personal hardships and disappointments. Not much ink has however been spilled on the actual problems and obstacles that émigré scientists encountered, when arriving and adapting to their new host countries. In examining the processes of scientific and cultural adaptation of some of these émigré researchers and physicians, when they arrived in their receiving cultures in North America, the articles in this special issue shift the local, primarily German-speaking context in neurology and psychiatry to the greater international level and the long-term effects since the 1930s and 1940s, along with their contributions to the emergence of interdisciplinarity in the new research field of neuroscience (including neurogenetics, biological psychiatry, and neuroimaging). Although such patterns identify sometimes preselective effects, not only of influential individuals— like the Frankfurt clinical neurologist Kurt Goldstein (1878–1965) or the Breslau psychiatric geneticist Franz Josef Kallmann (1897–1965)—or of local scientific milieus of the émigré neuroscientists, for example, at Harvard or Columbia University, these all had a decisive impact on the future development of the neurosciences during the 20th century.

Historiographical and methodological perspectives on the forced migration wave in twentieth-century neuroscience and psychiatry

In fact, the exodus of so many psychoanalysts, such as the Vienna-trained founder of modern psychosomatic medicine Franz Gabriel Alexander (1891–1964), who came to the University of Chicago, Frankfurt neurologist Leo Alexander (1905–1985), Sandor Radó (1890–1972) from Budapest, who went to Columbia University where he became the head of psychiatry, Helene Deutsch (1884–1982) from Vienna, who went to Boston and co-founded the Boston Psychoanalytic Institute, or the German émigré psychiatrist Charles Fischer (1902–1987) (later at the New York Psychoanalytic Institute), probably shaped North American neuropsychiatry, mental health, and experimental psychology in many more ways than any other process related to forced migration (Grob, 1983, pp. 124–165). With regard to the emerging interdisciplinary field of neuroscience in the German-speaking countries, our interest is rather on particular areas of biological psychiatry, such as the "emigration" of neurological synapse research, insulin-shock therapy, and neurogenetics. Their relationship with basic neuroscience brings the forced migration process closer in touch with the historiographical narrative of many of the articles assembled here. Some contradictory and fairly independent developments also become visible, since, for example, psychoanalysis became one of the major adversaries of shock therapies in the wider context of North American psychiatry and public mental health. The double *volte face* from the praise of psychoanalysis over brain psychiatry, its antagonism with genetic and biological psychiatry, and its later repulsion due to the advances in molecular medicine and clinical neuroscience was a ground-breaking process in the development of modern neuroscience in North America itself (Magoun, 2002, pp. 405–410).

According to American historian Jack Pressman's book *Last Resort: Psychosurgery and the Limits of Medicine* (1998), the reassessment and reevaluation of contemporary mental health practices towards the development of aggressive surgical and interventional psychiatric therapies was nevertheless already underway during the first half of the 1930s (Pressman, 1998, pp. 158–160). The new somatic forms of therapy had been particularly associated with Egaz Moniz' (1874–1955) psychosurgery in Lisbon, Portugal, and Ugo Cerletti (1877–1963) at La Sapienza University of Rome, where he developed electroconvulsion therapy (ECT) that became further adapted as Insulin- and Cardiazol-shock therapy later on. Among the émigrés, who were helped by the first group of transatlantic travelers, were major representatives of non-analytical brain psychiatry, such as psychiatric geneticist Franz Kallmann from Berlin and pioneers of somatic treatment approaches, for example, Ukraine-born and Vienna-trained neurophysiologist Manfred Sakel (1900–1957) as well as Budapest's Ladislaus von Meduna (1896–1964), who later joined their colleagues in major North American research centers in New York City and Chicago. Their examples clearly emphasize the important role played by the scientific intermediaries and often matching institutions. This early integrative process became further amplified through institutional involvements of the Rockefeller Foundation since 1934/1935, and its close ties to the German research institutions since the Weimar

Republic, as well as the American Emergency Committee in Aid of Displaced Foreign Scholars, which counted various German-born scientists among their members (Ash & Soellner, 1996, pp. 86–114).

Published disciplinary histories and available oral history accounts by scientific refugees have already pointed to major scientific achievements and methodological landmark events. The contributions of these refugees can be further analyzed through looking at the alignment of émigré neuroscientists with respective research groups involved in such developments as laboratory progress in neural regeneration research, new classifying approaches of brain tumor pathology, or the introduction of electron microscopy in histological nerve cell research, to name only a few. When prudently aligning this historiographical analysis with the development of early interdisciplinary approaches in German-speaking neuroscience, a number of very similar observations emerge as Israel-based historian Ute Deichmann has pointed out in her preceding work on emigration-induced changes in experimental biology: "The emigration of scientists after 1933 caused, with a higher probability, significant scientific change within novel fields of research rather than within the established ones" (Deichmann, 1996, p. 9).

The contributions to this issue of the *Journal of the History of the Neurosciences*

Bernd Holdorff's (Berlin) article, entitled "Emigrated Neuroscientists from Berlin to North America" begins this volume by describing the situation in Germany in 1933 when the Nazis rose to power. With the "Law on the Re-Establishment of the Professional Civil Service" being inaugurated in April of the same year, dozens of neurologists, brain psychiatrists, and neuropathologists were driven out of their university or city hospital positions in Berlin. This article describes the fate of several individuals in more detail, such as Frederic Henry Lewey, Kurt Goldstein, or Fred Quadfasel, while also concentrating on the specific collective biographical aspect of this emigration process. The second article by Stephen Pow (Budapest) and Frank W. Stahnisch (Calgary) is entitled "Eugenics Ideals, Racial Hygiene, and the Emigration Process of German-American Neurogeneticist Franz Josef Kallmann (1897–1965)." It looks at the career development of one of the most influential neurological and psychiatric geneticists of the 20th century, first in Germany and later in his North American exile. While Kallmann was largely successful in re-establishing his research program at the Department of Psychiatry at Columbia University's Medical School, this case example allows interesting insights into the relation-ship of competing research traditions by émigré clinical neuroscientists and psychiatrists, particularly the impact of the adherents of psychoanalysis on the early fate of biological psychiatry in the United States. The next article is coauthored by Lawrence A. Zeidman (Chicago), Anna von Villiez, Jan-Patrick Stellmann, and Hendrik van den Bussche (all from Hamburg) as "'History Had Taken Such a Large Piece Out of my Life' — Neuroscientist Refugees from Hamburg during National Socialism." Similar to the fore-going contributions, the article argues that 400 doctors in Hamburg alone were dismissed for their Jewish family background or political inclinations, while following the specific émigré biographies of 16 of them who had been faculty members before. The next contribution by Frank W. Stahnisch (Calgary), titled "Learning Soft Skills the Hard Way: Historiographical Considerations on the Cultural Adjustment Process of German-

Speaking Émigré Neuroscientists in Canada, 1933 to 1963," considers the typologies of the émigré neuropathologists Karl Stern (1906–1975), Robert Weil (1909–2002), and Heinz Lehmann (1911–1999). It thus complements the descriptions in the first three articles, which focus particularly on the United States as the receiving country, by emphasizing the local living and working situations of émigré researchers and academics in Canada. In her exceptionally innovative and extraordinary article, Gül Russell (College Station) focuses on a hitherto rather neglected group of émigré neurologists, neuropathologists, and brain psychiatrists, who under the aegis of German-Jewish neuropathologist Philipp Schwartz (1894–1977) found refuge and a second home in Turkey. Turkey, already influenced by the Humboldtian ideal of the German research university, benefited greatly from the group of German refugee professors and doctors in the development of its research institutions as well as the Turkish health care system at large. Her article is titled "A Variation on Forced Migration: Wilhelm Peters (Prussia via Britain to Turkey) and Muzafer Sherif (Turkey to the United States)." Turning to further special cases in the history of forced migration in the neurosciences, Aleksandra Loewenau (Calgary) thematizes in the final article "Between Resentment and Aid: German and Austrian Psychiatrist and Neurologist Refugees in Great Britain since 1933," the great many difficulties that these individuals faced when first trying to find continuing employment on the British Isles during the Second World War. Many of the psychiatrist and neurologist refugees, who are discussed in her article, then tried to migrate onwards to North America and other continents after the war. Loewenau's article thereby provides intriguing insights into Great Britain as a destination of permanent yet also transient exile for German-speaking émigré neuroscientists since 1933. Our special issue ends with a historiographical commentary from Delia Gavrus (Winnipeg), entitled "Émigré Scientists and the Global Turn in the History of Science: A Commentary on the Special Issue 'New Perspectives on Forced Migration in the History of Twentieth-Century Neuroscience,'" which situates the articles assembled in this issue in the wider discourse about emigration, international relationships, and biomedical progress in the recent history of medicine and science literature.

References

American Academy of Neurology (AAN) (1948–1953): Archives and Rare Books Division of the Becker Library, WUSM (PC053, records of the AAN, Series 7, history committee files, Box 3, folder: Historical materials, 1948–1953, lists of committees). St. Louis, MO, AAN.

Ash M, Soellner A, eds. (1996): *Forced Migration and Scientific Change: Émigré German–speaking Scientists after 1933*. Cambridge, Cambridge University Press.

Bleker J (1989): "Der Erfolg der Gleichschaltungsaktion kann als durchschlagend bezeichnet werden." Der Bund Deutscher Aerztinnen 1933–1936. In: Bleker J, Jachertz N, eds., *Medizin im "Dritten Reich."* Cologne, Deutscher Aerzteverlag, pp. 83–96.

Deichmann U (1996): *Biologists under Hitler*. Cambridge, MA, Harvard University Press.

Grob GN (1983): *Mental Illness and American Society: 1875–1940*. Princeton, NJ, Princeton University Press.

Herrn R (2010): "Magnus Hirschfeld, sein Institut fuer Sexualwissenschaft und die Buecherverbrennung." In Herrn R, ed., *Verfemt und Verboten: Vorgeschichte und Folgen der Buecherverbrennungen 1933.* Hildesheim, Olms–Verlag, pp. 97–152.

Holdorff B, Winau R, eds. (2001): *Geschichte der Neurologie in Berlin*. Berlin, DeGruyter.

Juette R (1990): *Die Emigration der deutschsprachigen 'Wissenschaft des Judentums'. Die Auswanderung juedischer Historiker nach Palaestina 1933–1945*. Stuttgart, Franz Steiner.

Kater K (1989): *Doctors under Hitler*. Chapel Hill, The University of North Carolina Press.

Krohn CD, von zur Muehlen P, Gerhard P, Winckler L, eds. (1998): *Handbuch der deutschsprachigen Emigration 1933–1945*. Darmstadt, Wissenschaftliche Verlagsbuchhandlung, Volume 3.

Longerich P (2010): *Holocaust: The Nazi Persecution and Murder of the Jews*. Oxford, Oxford University Press.

Magoun HW (2002): *American Neuroscience in the Twentieth Century: Confluence of the Neural, Behavioral, and Communicative Streams*, Marshall Louise H., ed. and annotated. Lisse, A. A. Balkema Publishers.

Medawar J, Pyke D (2001): *Hitler's Gift: The True Story of the Scientists Expelled by the Nazi Regime*. New York, Arkade Publishing.

Niederland D (1988): The emigration of Jewish Academics and professionals from Germany in the first years of Nazi rule. *Leo Baeck Institute Yearbook* 33: 285–300.

Pearle KM (1981): *Preventive Medicine: The Refugee Physicians and the New York Medical Community 1933–1945*, Working Papers on Blocked Alternatives in the Health Policy System. University of Bremen, Bremen.

Pressman JD (1998): *Last Resort: Psychosurgery and the Limits of Medicine*. Cambridge, Cambridge University Press.

Schwartz P (1995): *Notgemeinschaft: Zur Emigration deutscher Wissenschaftler in die Tuerkei*, Peukert H, ed. Metropolis, Marburg.

Stahnisch FW (2010): German-speaking émigré-neuroscientists in North America after 1933: Critical reflections on emigration-induced scientific change. *Oesterreichische Zeitschrift fuer Geschichtswissenschaften (Vienna)* 21: 36–68.

Strauss HA, Roeder W, eds. (1983): *International Biographical Dictionary of Central European Emigrés 1933–1945*. The Arts, Sciences, and Literature. 2 Volumes. Munich, K. G. Saur.

Weindling PJ (1989): *Health, Race and German Politics between National Unification and Nazism, 1870–1945*. Cambridge, Cambridge University Press.

Zeidman LA, Kondziella D (2012): Neuroscience in Nazi Europe: Victims of the Third Reich. *Canadian Journal of Neurological Sciences* 39: 729–746.

Zimmerman D (2006): The Society for the Protection of Science and Learning and the politicization of British science in the 1930s. *Minerva* 44: 25–45.

"History had taken such a large piece out of my life" — Neuroscientist refugees from Hamburg during National Socialism

Lawrence A. Zeidman, Anna von Villiez, Jan-Patrick Stellmann, and Hendrik van den Bussche

ABSTRACT

Approximately 9,000 physicians were uprooted for so-called "racial" or "political" reasons by the Nazi regime and 6,000 fled Germany. These refugees are often seen as survivors who contributed to a "brain drain" from Germany. About 432 doctors (all specialties, private and academic) were dismissed from the major German city of Hamburg. Of these, 16 were Hamburg University faculty members dismissed from their government-supported positions for "racial" reasons, and, of these, five were neuroscientists. In a critical analysis, not comprehensively done previously, we will demonstrate that the brain drain did not equal a "brain gain." The annihilation of these five neuroscientists' careers under different but similar auspices, their shameful harassment and incarceration, financial expropriation by Nazi ransom techniques, forced migration, and roadblocks once reaching destination countries stalled and set back any hopes of research and quickly continuing once-promising careers. A major continuing challenge is finding ways to repair an open wound and obvious vacuum in the German neuroscience community created by the largely collective persecution of colleagues 80 years ago.

Introduction

With regard to Nazi persecution of "non-Aryan" (Jewish) and leftist neuroscientists,[1] what is the significance of Hamburg and why focus an article on this major German city? First, a comprehensive case study on the tragic "de-Jewification" (removal of Jews, in Nazi parlance) of Hamburg neurologists and psychiatrists has not been published before,

---

Color versions of one or more of the figures in the article can be found online at www.tandfonline.com/njhn.

[1] With respect to the retrospective analysis, many of the individuals in this article are anachronistically referred to collectively as "neuroscientists," though that term did not emerge until the 1960s with the creation of the Neurosciences Research Program in which experts in neurology, psychiatry, and other related basic biomedical fields met to confront ongoing research challenges in an interdisciplinary fashion (see Adelman, 1987). Additionally, neurology and psychiatry were typically linked in Germany until after World War II, separating when diagnostic and therapeutic advancements in neurology made it distinct and viable enough as a specialty to practice separately (see Janzen, 1977; Holdorff, 2004).

especially not in English. Secondly, Hamburg hosted a relatively large group of Jewish neuroscientists (see below). Thirdly, Hamburg was of special interest in the Nazi era because the town featured one of the most important neurological clinics in the Reich and one of the few independent chairs in neurology at Hamburg-Eppendorf University Hospital, originally led by Max Nonne (1860–1959), and from 1935 on by NSDAP[2] member Heinrich Pette (1887–1964).[3] Pette was Deputy *Reichsleiter* [Reich Leader] for neurology in the *Gesellschaft deutscher Neurologen und Psychiater* [Society of German Neurologists and Psychiatrists], the forcibly merged organization of the formerly separate neurology and psychiatry societies in the Nazi era (Schmuhl, 2011).

While a detailed discussion of Hamburg neuroscience's *Gleichschaltung* (Nazi subordination) and its ramifications is outside the scope of this article, we will outline the general persecution measures against non-Aryan physicians in Nazi Germany and in Hamburg neurology and describe the fate of five academic Jewish neuroscientists dismissed from their positions in Hamburg: Hermann Josephy (later Herman: 1887–1960), Walter Rudolf Kirschbaum (1894–1982), Victor Kafka (1881–1955), Friedrich Wohlwill (1881–1958), and Richard Loewenberg (1898–1954). Many common and unique issues were faced by these five, and we will describe their personal and professional ramifications. We obtained the names of the dismissed Hamburg neuroscientists from two extensively researched studies in German two of us have already conducted on medical care in Hamburg in the "Third Reich" (von Villiez, 2009; van den Bussche, 2014a). The information from these books was supplemented with new data from files located at the Hamburg Staatsarchiv [Hamburg State Archive], Hamburg University History Library (Arbeitsstelle und Bibliothek fuer Universitaetsgeschichte), Norwegian Riksarkivet, Swedish Riksarkivet, the Society of the Protection of Science and Learning (SPSL) collection in Oxford, Archives of the Chicago Neurological Society, U.S. National Archives, and personal communications with the European historian and psychoanalyst Peter Loewenberg (b. 1933) at the University of California in Los Angeles (son of Richard Loewenberg).

The "Aryanization" of Hamburg neuroscience

Of 432 Hamburg physicians (all specialties) professionally persecuted (i.e., fired or removed from insurance panels) under the Nazis (von Villiez, 2009), 19 Hamburg University medical faculty (Professors and *Privatdozenten* [lecturers or adjunct professors]) were dismissed for racial or political reasons (the other 413 were private practitioners). Of these 19 academics, 16 (84%) were dismissed as "non-Aryan," and three were forced into early retirement (van den Bussche, 2014a). The five neuroscientists we discuss below were thus representative of the largest group of persecuted academic physicians.

"De-Jewification" was a stepwise marginalization of Jewish physicians in the form of "legal" and illegal professional, financial, and physical persecutory measures, but these victims also experienced postemigration tribulations. Relentless professional legislation against Jews (including "partial-Jews" and Aryans married with non-Aryans) began soon

---

[2]*Nationalsozialistische Deutsche Arbeiterpartei* (National Socialist German Workers' Party; the Nazi Party).
[3]Hamburg Staatsarchiv (Henceforth listed as "StAHH") 361-6_I_319 Personalakte: Pette, Heinrich.

after the Nazi *Machtergreifung* ("power seizure") in January 1933. First, Jewish civil servant physicians and university professors and lecturers were dismissed under Paragraph 3 of the so-called Law for the Reestablishment of the German Civil Service (*Gesetz zur Wiederherstellung des Berufsbeamtentums*) of April 7, 1933 (Proctor, 1988). Political dissidents (e.g., communists and "pacifists") were also included in this massive Nazi "cleansing" (Paragraph 4; Proctor, 1988; Kater, 1989a, 1989b). Their posts were taken over by young "Aryans" (Shevell, 1999; Stahnisch, 2010). Those dismissed under Paragraphs 3 and 4 of the law should generally not receive a pension unless they had served in the role for at least 10 years (Paragraph 8). With Paragraph 6, individuals could be forcibly retired without cause to "simplify administration … even if they are not yet incapacitated." All of those dismissed were to be removed from office by September 30, 1933 (Anonymous, 1933). Some received transient protection from the dismissals with so-called "Hindenburg exemptions," mainly applying to doctors who were frontline World War One (WWI) fighters (Kater, 1989b). These physicians were allowed to continue their private or insurance practice for the time being. Most exemptions ended with the 1935 Nuernberg Laws, with which all full Jews lost their Reich citizenship and became merely German "residents" (Proctor, 1988).

The penultimate Jewish medical disfranchisement occurred on July 25, 1938, with a new law decertifying Jewish doctors by October (Kater, 1989b). Three thousand Jewish doctors remained in Germany in 1938, and only 700 were allowed to provide basic health care to the remaining Jews as *Krankenbehandlern* (derogatory term: health practitioners) (Barkai, 2000). Besides the professional and academic persecution faced by Jewish neuroscientists, another type was financial persecution to fill the coffers of the Nazi state. In 1933, the total property of German Jews was about 16 Billion Reichsmarks (RM), of which a quarter was safely brought into exile. But the Nazis aimed to gain the rest (Kuller, 2004), through different taxes: the *Judenvermoegensabgabe* [property tax],[4] the emigration tax (Reich Flight Tax, *Reichsfluchtsteuer*) (Kater, 1989b), and the DEGO-Tax on any item acquired for emigration.[5] Thus, at the height of Jewish desperation to emigrate in 1938–1939 before the war, the Nazis claimed nearly all of their assets prior to departure, collecting about 900 million RM total by 1940 (Kater, 1989b). Already, they had stolen 1.1 billion RM with the *Judenvermoegensabgabe* (Kuller, 2004).

Physical and psychological persecution took the form of sanctioned arrest and imprisonment and torture. It was generally not illegal to victimize Jews in the Nazi state, and they lived in a precarious state of "legality" in which harassment was condoned by the Nazified judiciary (Kater, 1989b). Beside boycotts, random terror by Nazi stormtroopers and arrests for trumped-up charges by the Gestapo (Nazi secret state police) affected non-Aryan doctors. The culmination of this violence was the well-orchestrated Nazi pogroms in November 1938, called *Kristallnacht* [Night of Broken Glass] throughout Germany. Many Jewish doctors were arrested on sight and deported to a concentration camp (Kater, 1989b). They were released if they agreed to "emigrate" and release their property to the Nazi state. "De-Jewification" of German medicine resulted in up to 9,000 Jewish and "politically unreliable" doctors losing their positions in Germany (Kater, 1989b; Stahnisch, 2010), with the majority emigrating but at least 2,000 murdered, most in the later Holocaust, and some 450 committing suicide (Zeidman & Kondziella, 2012).

---

[4]*Verordnung ueber eine Suehneleistung der Juden deutscher Staatsangehoerigkeit* (RGBl. I S. 1579). November 12, 1938.
[5]DEGO-Tax was a payment to the *Deutsche Golddiskontbank* (Barkai, 2000).

Five dismissed academic neuroscientists

Hermann Josephy

Hermann Josephy (see Fig. 1), born in Schwaan, Germany, was a Jewish neurologist and neuropathologist who after serving as a WWI combatant, began psychiatric work under Alfons Jakob (1884–1931; codescriber of Creutzfeldt-Jakob disease [CJD]; Sammet, 2008), in Hamburg-Friedrichsberg State Mental Hospital. He obtained his Hamburg University psychiatry habilitation in 1924 and the title of *nichtbeamteter ausserordentlicher Professor* (nonpermanent associate professor [nbaoP]) in 1930. After Jakob's death, Josephy became the leader of the Neuroanatomy Department (Prosector) in 1932. But Josephy lost his teaching permit and his position by November 1933 since he was "non-Aryan."[6] As a loophole measure had given Josephy's veteran status, he was actually dismissed under Paragraph 6 of the Reconstitution Law (see Fig. 2).[7] Josephy was replaced in 1937 at Friedrichsberg by the 30-year-old "Aryan" Hans Jacob (1907–1997),[8] who that same year became an NSDAP member.[9] Josephy started private practice and continued working at the Hamburg Israelite Hospital until 1938. He also gave a series of neuropathology lectures at the University of Copenhagen in 1934 and at the Hebrew University of Jerusalem in 1937.[10]

But private practice and a meager state pension did not provide enough income.[11] Josephy received a reference letter from Friedrichsberg Hospital Director Wilhelm Weygandt (1870–1939) and initially applied for help in October 1933 to the Academic Assistance Council (AAC) in England, followed much later by an application to the

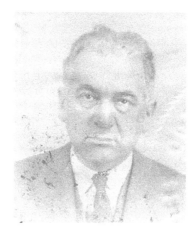

Figure 1. Hermann Josephy. National Archives and Records Administration (NARA), Great Lakes Division, Chicago, IL. Public Domain.

---

[6]Oxford Bodleian SPSL file 395-5: Josephy, Hermann.
[7]StAHH 131-11-1567: Hermann Josephy.
[8]Ibid.
[9]StAHH 361-6_IV_1877: PA Jacob, Hans.
[10]Oxford Bodleian SPSL file 395-5: Josephy, Hermann.
[11]File from the "Devisenstelle" of the "Oberfinanzpraesident Hamburg", Sta HH/OFP 314-15/F1204.

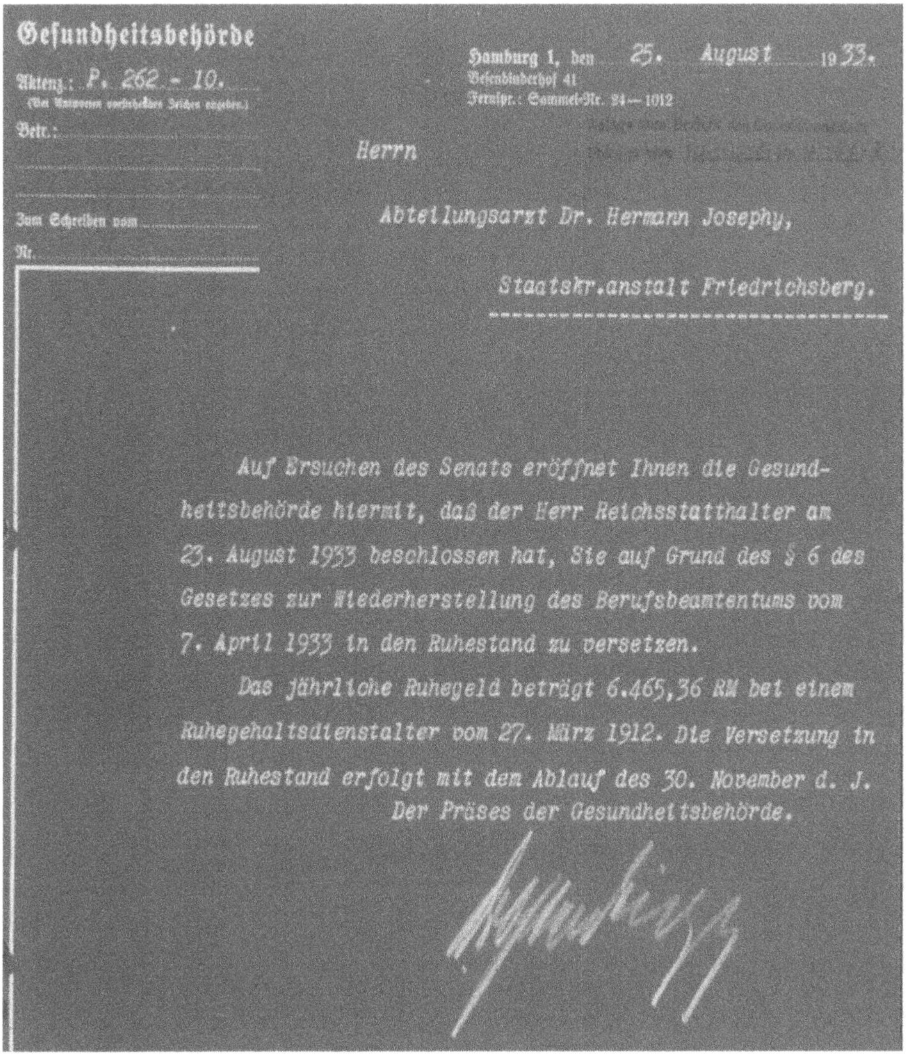

Gesundheitsbehörde
Aktenz.: P. 262 - 10.
(Bei Antworten vorstehendes Zeichen angeben.)
Betr.:
Zum Schreiben vom
Nr.

Hamburg 1, den 25. August 1933.
Besenbinderhof 41
Fernspr.: Sammel-Nr. 24—1012

Herrn

Abteilungsarzt Dr. Hermann Josephy,

Staatskr.anstalt Friedrichsberg.

Auf Ersuchen des Senats eröffnet Ihnen die Gesundheitsbehörde hiermit, daß der Herr Reichsstatthalter am 23. August 1933 beschlossen hat, Sie auf Grund des § 6 des Gesetzes zur Wiederherstellung des Berufsbeamtentums vom 7. April 1933 in den Ruhestand zu versetzen.

Das jährliche Ruhegeld beträgt 6.465,36 RM bei einem Ruhegehaltsdienstalter vom 27. März 1912. Die Versetzung in den Ruhestand erfolgt mit dem Ablauf des 30. November d. J.

Der Präses der Gesundheitsbehörde.

Figure 2. Dismissal notice under Paragraph 6 of the Reconstitution Law for Josephy (StAHH 131-11-1567, Josephy, p. 20). © Hamburg Staatsarchiv.

AAC-successor Society for Protection of Science and Learning (SPSL, changed in 1936) in England in December 1938.[12] Josephy's connections in Copenhagen were not fruitful enough to make an escape possible and, despite his lectures in Jerusalem,[13] staying in Palestine (present-day Israel) was not possible as Palestine did not need more academic specialists. The British government restricted the number of Jewish immigrants fearing an uprising and collaboration of the Arabic population with Nazi Germany (Barkai, 2000).

[12]Oxford Bodleian SPSL file 395-5: Josephy, Hermann.
[13]Ibid.

During *Kristallnacht*, Josephy was deported to the Sachsenhausen concentration camp for more than a month.[14] He was released when his wife presented documents proving their intended flight to America.[15] The Josephys obtained visas and immigrated in April 1939 to Britain, where a friend had financially vouched for them[16]; the guarantor in Britain was necessary to obtain the British visa, despite a job offer in Chicago, an affidavit from a wealthy friend in Chicago, and support from the SPSL, since the Josephys had been forced to liquidate most of their assets to pay Nazi taxes.[17] In the United Kingdom, Josephy first had an unpaid research position at the Cardiff City Mental Hospital in the laboratory of brain metabolism researcher Juda Quastel (1899–1987), who had an interest in Josephy's neurological research.[18] His next position was at Runwell Hospital in Essex.[19] Josephy's plan was to temporarily wait in Britain for his visa to the United States, where he had been offered an internship at Michael Reese Hospital (MRH) in Chicago.[20] Josephy could not obtain a "non-quota" US visa because he had not taught for two years, thus he had to queue on the quota list.[21] From May to September 1940, Josephy was interned with other "C" class aliens[22] in Britain.[23] In October 1940, Josephy and his wife finally qualified for American visas and immigrated to Illinois.[24] Due to his late arrival in America, Josephy was not able to take the MRH internship. He also passed the state board examination in 1941, which he hoped would allow him to progress from his "modest position" in central Illinois in a state mental institute for the "feebleminded," the Lincoln State School and Colony, to a "good position." Indeed, in 1945 he became laboratory director at the 4,500-bed Chicago State Hospital, a mental institute, finally practicing as a neuropathologist again. However, the salary there was also inadequate, his wife worked as a technician in the hospital, and they lived on the hospital premises, thus to Josephy this situation was merely "satisfactory."[25] From 1949–1952, Josephy became an Associate Professor at the Chicago Medical School (Anonymous, 1960).

Walter Rudolf Kirschbaum

Walter Rudolf Kirschbaum (see Fig. 3), born in Duisburg, Germany, served in WWI in the artillery and as a medical officer but finished his medical studies in 1919 after training in neurology at Berlin's Charité Hospital (1916–1918) and the Berlin-Moabit Institute of Pathology. He was Assistant under Weygandt and Jakob at Hamburg-

---

[14]Information courtesy of the Stiftung Brandenburgische Gedenkstaetten/Gedenkstaette und Museum Sachsenhausen. Original file located at: Russian State Military Archive, Moscow 1367/1/20, Bl. 070.
[15]Oxford Bodleian SPSL file 395-5: Josephy, Hermann.
[16]Ibid.
[17]File from the "Devisenstelle" of the "Oberfinanzpräsident Hamburg," StAHH/OFP 314-15/F1204.
[18]Oxford Bodleian SPSL Home Office file 433-4: Josephy, Hermann.
[19]Oxford Bodleian SPSL file 395-5: Josephy, Hermann
[20]Oxford Bodleian SPSL Home Office file 433-4: Josephy, Hermann.
[21]Ibid.
[22]C-class German and Austrian aliens in Britain were theoretically supposed to have protection from internment, given that they were refugees from Nazi oppression. But men living in a "protected area" could be arrested and interned. See: Oxford Bodleian SPSL file 395-5: Josephy, Hermann.
[23]Oxford Bodleian SPSL file 395-5: Josephy, Hermann.
[24]Ibid.
[25]Ibid.

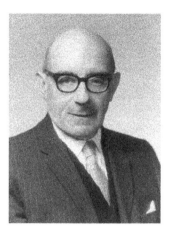

Figure 3. Walter R. Kirschbaum, MD, unknown year. © Archives of the Chicago Neurological Society, Boshes Library of the Neurosciences, University of Illinois at Chicago Department of Neurology and Rehabilitation.

Friedrichsberg beginning in 1921 and in 1927 was made an *Oberarzt* [senior consultant]. By 1933, he became *Privatdozent* with a habilitation on psychosis in neurosyphilis.[26] Kirschbaum had already published a pioneering study on encephalitis lethargica for his doctoral dissertation in 1919, and, in 1924, he published on two autosomal dominant hereditary CJD cases.[27] But in 1934, despite 32 publications and a burgeoning career, Kirschbaum's *Privatdozent* title was revoked because of his non-Aryan descent; like Josephy, he lost his position under the loophole Paragraph 6 of the Reconstitution Law (see Fig. 4).[28]

Kirschbaum applied to the AAC but only received an offer in South Africa that eventually did not materialize.[29] Thereafter, he continued a limited private practice in his apartment until 1938.[30] Like Josephy, Kirschbaum was imprisoned at the Sachsenhausen concentration camp after *Kristallnacht* but was released three weeks earlier than Josephy[31]; Kirschbaum was assisted "strenuously" by his Christian wife.[32] Kirschbaum immigrated directly to Chicago in 1939. Except for a special permit for his "Aryan" wife to export her jewelry,[33] Kirschbaum had to leave all financial properties in Germany and restart life in America as an exploited refugee.

In Chicago, Kirschbaum completed an internship at MRH and in 1940 obtained his Illinois medical license. He then worked at Manteno State Hospital in Joliet

---

[26]Oxford Bodleian SPSL file 395-9: Kirschbaum, Walter.
[27]Ibid.
[28]StAHH 361-6 IV 1200.
[29]Oxford Bodleian SPSL file 395-9: Kirschbaum, Walter.
[30]Ibid.
[31]Information courtesy of the Stiftung Brandenburgische Gedenkstaetten/Gedenkstaette und Museum Sachsenhausen. Original file located at: Russian State Military Archive, Moskow 1367/1/15, Bl. 077 and 1367/1/20, Bl. 135.
[32]Kirschbaum WR. Letter to Dr. Louis Boshes, June 12, 1970. Archives of the Chicago Neurological Society. Boshes Library of the Neurosciences. University of Illinois at Chicago (UIC) Neuropsychiatric Institute, Chicago, IL, USA.
[33]File from the "Devisenstelle" of the "Oberfinanzpräsident Hamburg", StAHH/OFP 314-15/F1299.

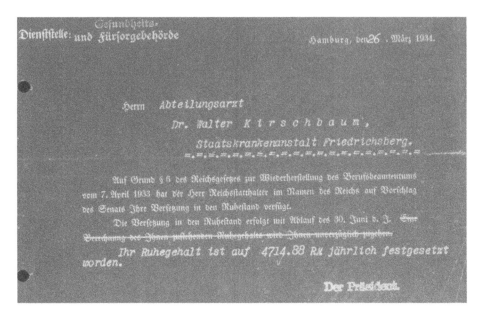

Figure 4. Dismissal notice under Paragraph 6 of the Reconstitution Law for Kirschbaum (StAHH 361-6 IV 1200, Kirschbaum, p. 6). © Hamburg Staatsarchiv.

(1940–1947), first as a pathologist and then as a ward physician, helping with malaria research during the war. He received a better home on hospital grounds for his later work but was dissatisfied overall with the lack of research opportunities there.[34] Kirschbaum joined Northwestern University's Neurology Department as an unsalaried Assistant Professor in 1948 but continued to need part-time Veterans Administration (VA) Hospital work and his private practice to support his family. He became an attending physician at Cook County Hospital in 1952 and was appointed Neurology Chairman there later.[35] Reflecting on his career, Kirschbaum stated, "History had taken such a large piece out of my life. I felt I could not waste time and I worked hard."[36] Kirschbaum eventually became an *Extraordinarius* (Associate Professor) of neurology in 1957 at Hamburg University in the course of his reparation request.[37] He also became Associate Professor (and later Emeritus) at Northwestern in 1958.[38] Kirschbaum published at least 22 articles and book chapters in exile.[39] Late in his career, Kirschbaum collected all the CJD cases he could find and

[34]Kirschbaum WR. Letter to Dr. Louis Boshes, June 12, 1970. Archives of the Chicago Neurological Society. Boshes Library of the Neurosciences. UIC Neuropsychiatric Institute, Chicago, IL, USA.

[35]Ibid.

[36]Ibid.

[37]Files of the Medical Faculty of Hamburg University, file Kirschbaum (without file number).

[38]Boshes LD. In Memoriam: Dr. Walter R. Kirschbaum, 1894–1982. Archives of the Chicago Neurological Society. Boshes Library of the Neurosciences. UIC Neuropsychiatric Institute, Chicago, IL, USA. pp. 1–5; Kirschbaum WR. Curriculum Vitae, March 12, 1958. Archives of the Chicago Neurological Society. Boshes Library of the Neurosciences. UIC Neuropsychiatric Institute, Chicago, IL, USA.

[39]Ibid.

wrote a book summarizing the first 150 (Kirschbaum, 1968).[40] Regarding his CJD book, Kirschbaum lamented, "It is a late endeavor and I hope a successful one. I feel I have not begun to fulfill the expectations which my teachers and colleagues in Germany once had for me."[41]

Victor Kafka

Victor Kafka (see Fig. 5), born in Karlsbad, Austro-Hungary (then Czechoslovakia after WWI and modern-day Czech Republic), was an Evangelical Lutheran but of Jewish descent.[42] He was a psychiatry assistant at Prague's German University before moving to Hamburg in 1911 to join the Friedrichsberg Psychiatric Clinic.[43] In 1915, he founded and headed the Chemical-Bacteriological-Serological Department there since 1920. By 1926, he became *Oberarzt* at Friedrichsberg and *Privatdozent* in 1919 at Hamburg University, followed by nbaoP for psychiatry by 1924. He was a pioneer and expert in cerebrospinal fluid (CSF) analysis and had 182 publications from 1906– 1934 mainly on CSF pathophysiology and diagnostics in neurosyphilis, epilepsy, meningitis, and brain tumors.[44] His book *The Cerebrospinal Fluid* (Kafka, 1930) in his words was a "standard work," and his earlier *Pocketbook of the Practical Methods of Investigation for Nervous and Mental Diseases* (Kafka, 1917) had four editions.[45]

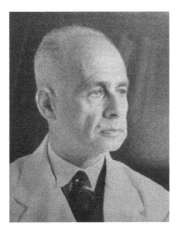

Figure 5. Victor Kafka (Demme, 1951). Dr. Hans Demme of Hamburg, presumed owner of the photo and copyright holder per Springer Publications (since no source listed for the photo in the original article), died in 1964.

---

[40]Boshes LD. In Memoriam: Dr. Walter R. Kirschbaum, 1894–1982. Archives of the Chicago Neurological Society. Boshes Library of the Neurosciences. UIC Neuropsychiatric Institute, Chicago, IL, USA. pp. 1–5.
[41]Kirschbaum WR. Letter to Dr. Louis Boshes, June 12, 1970. Archives of the Chicago Neurological Society. Boshes Library of the Neurosciences. UIC Neuropsychiatric Institute, Chicago, IL, USA.
[42]Oxford Bodleian SPSL file 395-6: Kafka, Victor.
[43]Ibid.
[44]Ibid.
[45]Ibid.

Per his student, neurologist Hans Demme (1900–1964), "he did not connect easily to other people" (Demme, 1951, p. 361), perhaps explaining why only 15 of 182 publications were co-authored with others, such as one with Kirschbaum (Kafka & Kirschbaum, 1922).[46] Kafka did help his assistants publish 35 articles separately, including a 1930 article by Demme on the CSF protein ratio in neurological diseases (Demme, 1930). In 1928, Kafka became president of the Greater Hamburg Society of Neurologists and Psychiatrists.[47]

Despite international eminence and a still active career, Kafka was dismissed as *Oberarzt* in June 1933.[48] In July 1933, he was notified that by the end of the year he would lose his professorship under Paragraph 6 of the Reconstitution Law. Kafka was not entitled to a pension despite being *Oberarzt* for over 10 years, possibly because he was not a WWI combatant. Kafka was forced to work in private practice. He still managed to publish another nine articles through 1939 despite his tribulations, and he lectured informally to Hamburg Jewish doctors and dentists from 1934–1939 and to Warsaw doctors in 1937.[49] He initially applied to the AAC July 12, 1933, but he did not send them his curriculum vitae, a testimonial from Weygandt, and his publication list until over a year later in October, 1934.[50] Despite his eminence and age on initial inquiry (under 60), Kafka did not find a position in Britain, possibly due to negative impressions on influential British neurologists such as Joseph Godwin Greenfield (1884–1958) from Queen's Square Hospital for Nervous Diseases:

> [Greenfield] appreciates Kafka's intellectual qualities, but on the personal side doubts whether he would fit into the Laboratory here ... he is inclined to be a little too aggressive and was not easy to work with.[51]

Given Greenfield's impression, other Queen Square neurologist Edward A. Carmichael (1896–1978) stated that "I feel, therefore, that it would be unwise to push his application here."[52] Kafka had written in desperate straits to Greenfield in April 1939 that he was still in Germany because the Czech quota for the United States was exhausted and he could not get a non-quota visa because the New York hospital that offered him a contract and medical school appointment did not have an official nursing school.[53]

In November 1935, Kafka had been arrested and imprisoned for over a month in the concentration camp Fuhlsbuettel in solitary confinement, like other Jews accused of a trumped-up charge of taking part in conversations that had disparaged the government,[54] but Kafka denied any political connections and decried the injustice.[55] Kafka lost his medical license in 1938 and became a *Krankenbehandler* by July 1939.[56] He immigrated with his wife to Oslo, Norway, in August 1939. Kafka had written to Nonne in 1939 asking

---

[46]Ibid.
[47]Ibid.
[48]StAHH 352-10 239 Hamburg Medizinalkollegium Personalakte, Victor Kafka.
[49]Oxford Bodleian SPSL file 395-6: Kafka, Victor.
[50]Ibid.
[51]Ibid., p. 304.
[52]Ibid.
[53]Oxford Bodleian SPSL file 395-6: Kafka, Victor.
[54]StAHH 352-10 239 Hamburg Medizinalkollegium Personalakte, Victor Kafka.
[55]Oxford Bodleian SPSL file 395-6: Kafka, Victor.
[56]StAHH 352-10 239 Hamburg Medizinalkollegium Personalakte, Victor Kafka.

him for possible job opportunities in Scandinavia, lamenting "How long will I and my wife be able to stand this."[57] In Oslo, Kafka worked at the *Statens institut for folkehelsa* [State institute for Public Health]; he founded a biological department there and became its leader.[58] Notably, Kafka was one of only 10 Jewish doctors employed by the Norwegian government in 1939/1940.[59] Despite persecution of Jews in Norway after the 1940 German occupation and Jewish deportations beginning in October 1942, Kafka remained in his post at institute director Einar Aaser's (1886–1976) request. Aaser tried to protect Kafka from personal molestation, calling him "absolutely indispensable"; this only succeeded until the end of November.[60,61] On December 2, 1942, with the ongoing Jewish deportations from Norway, Kafka made a risky escape to Sweden.[62] Kafka was aided in escape by journalist Tove Filseth (1905–1994) of the Norwegian resistance, who had helped large numbers of Jewish refugees escape (Cohen, 1997). Kafka was employed within weeks at the Långbro Sjukhus, a mental facility in Alvsjö, near Stockholm.[63,64]

Kafka attempted again to find a position in the United Kingdom in 1943, via help from the SPSL and British Council. The attempt was unsuccessful again.[65] He had to continually apply for renewed asylum and visas in Sweden, until the summer of 1944 when he acquired foreigner passports for himself and his wife, giving them traveling rights within nonrestricted areas of Sweden, but not Swedish citizenship.[66] Kafka was eventually granted a Swedish medical license in October 1947, followed by Swedish citizenship in January 1955.[67] Though he had no publications from 1940–1943 when his personal security was threatened in occupied Norway, he was able to publish 12 articles while in Sweden from 1943–1946.[68]

After the war, Kafka investigated the possibility of returning to Friedrichsberg in his old position; however, he was told that his age and the changed laboratory situation were obstacles. Eventually, he did come back to Hamburg and gave one or more lectures at the medical faculty.[69] His personal life was fractured, poignantly reflected by the fact that in 1951 his nationality was still listed as "stateless." His compensation claims resulted in some financial restitution by January 1955. But four months after obtaining Swedish citizenship and financial compensation from Germany, Kafka tragically died. Adding insult to injury, the full reparation amount was never paid to his widow.[70] Former NSDAP-member Demme, the *NS-Vertrauensmann* (Nazi "Steward") at Hamburg

---

[57]Kafka, V to Nonne, M, 16 May 1939, Hamburg State Archive, Nachlass M. Nonne (Peiffer, 2004, p. 555).
[58]Oxford Bodleian SPSL file 395-6: Kafka, Victor.
[59]Swedish Riksarkivet Archive File from the State Aliens Commission (Statens Utlänningskommission) on Victor Kafka.
[60]Ibid.
[61]Swedish Riksarkivet Archive. Files from the Swedish Ministry of Justice and the Ministry of Health and Social Affairs (Socialdepartementet) on Victor Kafka.
[62]Oxford Bodleian SPSL file 395-6: Kafka, Victor.
[63]Ibid.
[64]Swedish Riksarkivet Archive. Files from the Swedish Ministry of Justice and the Ministry of Health and Social Affairs (Socialdepartementet) on Victor Kafka.
[65]Oxford Bodleian SPSL file 395-6: Kafka, Victor.
[66]Swedish Riksarkivet Archive File from the State Aliens Commission (Statens Utlaenningskommission) on Victor Kafka.
[67]Swedish Riksarkivet Archive Files from the Swedish Ministry of Justice and the Ministry of Health and Social Affairs (Socialdepartementet) on Victor Kafka.
[68]Ibid.
[69]StAHH 361-6 I 233: Kafka medical faculty personnel file.
[70]StAHH 351-11 12215: Wiedergutmachungsakte Kafka.

University Medical School (van den Bussche, 2014a), who in 1934 had eagerly replaced a dismissed Jewish neurologist to become neurology director at the General Hospital Hamburg-Barmbek (Pieper, 2003), wrote a seventieth birthday tribute to his former teacher, stating that Kafka "was heavily burdened with the fact he was uprooted from his work" and how challenging it was "to overcome the difficulties mounting in front of him." Demme expressed gratitude "for the human interest" Kafka had in his pupils' fates and stated "May he be blessed with a long and beneficial time for work" (Demme, 1951, p. 361). It is an embarrassment that Demme failed to take responsibility publicly and to apologize for his and his Nazi colleagues' assistance in Hamburg's "de-Jewification" and curtailing of Kafka's highly productive career.

Friedrich Wohlwill

Friedrich Wohlwill (see Fig. 6), born in Hamburg, worked as a voluntary doctor and later Assistant in the University Pathological Institute at Hamburg-Eppendorf from 1905–1908, then worked as an assistant in Nonne's Clinical Department of Neurology until 1910. From 1910–1912, Wohlwill worked in the Halle University *Nervenklinik* (Neurology and Psychiatry Clinic). During these four years of clinical neurological activity, Wohlwill became primarily interested in neuropathology that would engage him for his entire career. After returning to Hamburg, he became a private neurologist and volunteer again at the Pathological Institute, especially examining the neurological material. During WWI, Wohlwill was an assistant again under Nonne in a military reserve hospital and then, in 1919, became Second Assistant at the Pathological Institute and later that year was habilitated at Hamburg University in pathological anatomy. Simultaneously with Kafka, Wohlwill became nbaoP in 1924 and the same year *Oberarzt* and Prosector at the *Allgemeines Krankenhaus* (General Hospital) St. Georg. In 1933 Wohlwill listed at least 62 of 127 (49%) articles first or coauthored as neuroscience related.[71]

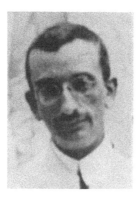

Figure 6. Friedrich Wohlwill (van den Bussche, 1989). © Hendrik van den Bussche of Hamburg, Germany.

---

[71]Oxford Bodleian SPSL file 409-10: Wohlwill, Friedrich.

In July 1933 (see Fig. 7), Wohlwill was notified that by September he would be dismissed as a "non-Aryan" under Paragraph 3 of the Reconstitution Law.[72] He worked briefly as Prosector at the Hamburg Jewish Hospital[73] but applied to the AAC in November 1933. He stated that he was looking for a position as a Prosector in a pathological institute or possibly as director of a neuropathological institute.[74] In June 1934, Wohlwill left for Lisbon, Portugal, where he had received an offer at the Instituto de Oncologia (Cancer Institute) without AAC help. He established the pathological research institute there and was also Prosector, becoming known as the founder of the "German School of Pathology" in Portugal.[75] From October 1936, Wohlwill was Prosector at Lisbon University Hospital (St. Martha), and, from 1945, he was full professor of Pathology there (Andrae and van den Bussche, 1998). Wohlwill had been the teacher of many Portuguese medical students in

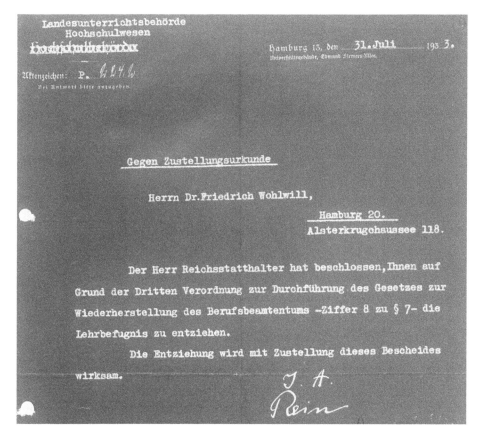

Figure 7. Dismissal notice under Paragraph 3 of the Reconstitution Law for Wohlwill (351-11-5442, Wohlwill, p. 4). © Hamburg Staatsarchiv.

---

[72]StAHH 351-11-5442 Wohlwill.
[73]StAHH 352-3 IV C70 Wohlwill.
[74]Oxford Bodleian SPSL file 409-10: Wohlwill, Friedrich.
[75]StAHH 352-3 IV C70 Wohlwill; StAHH 361-1 IV 1125 Wohlwill.

Hamburg and later they invited him to the Cancer Institute.[76] Also, like he did with Kafka, Nonne helped Wohlwill find the position in Lisbon. But Wohlwill lamented to Nonne that his uprooting and new position did not come close to equaling what he lost despite his expectations being low.[77] His working conditions at the Cancer Institute were poor. The new building was not finished, conditions for pathological examinations insufficient, the director acted like a "little dictator," whereby money was lacking and "as I am only a guest I cannot do anything [about] it."[78] Wohlwill had a five-year contract at the Cancer Institute but apparently was unable to obtain a Portuguese medical license and his income was entirely dependent on private tuition fees for lecturing to medical students. This income was not large but was "sufficient."[79]

In 1946, after 12 years in Portugal, Wohlwill emigrated to America where his children had previously emigrated because of lack of opportunities or fear of German invasion in Portugal.[80] Wohlwill found a job for six months at the M. J. Bassett Hospital in Cooperstown, New York, described by him as "a simple country hospital"[81] (Andrae and van den Bussche, 1998). From 1947, he worked at Danvers State Hospital in Hawthorne, Massachusetts.[82] His job there he described as "much less satisfying," his colleagues' interest in his work "equals 0" and he felt professionally "isolated and lonely."[83] He kept in touch with some former Jewish and "Aryan" colleagues in Germany, even writing a "*Persilschein*" [whitewash certificate][84] for former NSDAP member Hans Erhard Bock (1903–2004) (Klee, 2005). Despite dissatisfaction, Wohlwill worked at Danvers until 1952 because he was tired of resettling.[85] He was counting on a position at the Army Institute of Pathology that however did not materialize for unknown reasons.[86] Wohlwill was instead told to find a position in the VA in the South where a great pathologist deficiency existed, but he was not interested: "The local climate — both the geographical and the cultural — are not appealing to me."[87] Wohlwill had to leave Danvers in July 1952. Instead, he received an offer to become coinvestigator on a research project on nuclear energy at Boston University. Wohlwill stated that the Boston research job was temporary, "but in my age one has to be grateful to have work at all and we emigrants all live from hand to mouth more or less."[88] Despite that an alternative position at Harvard Medical School as Neuropathology Institute Consultant at the Warren Anatomical Museum, offered by neuropathologist Paul Yakovlev (1894–1983), had a lower salary than the Boston University one and, per Wohlwill, "the work ... suited me better" so he

[76]Oxford Bodleian SPSL file 409-410: Wohlwill, Friedrich.
[77]Number 1458, Wohlwill to Nonne, 28/12/1934, StAHH Nachlass M. Nonne (Peiffer, 2004, pp. 944–946).
[78]Ibid.
[79]Oxford Bodleian SPSL file 409-10: Wohlwill, Friedrich.
[80]StAHH 352-3 IV C70 Friedrich Wohlwill.
[81]StAHH 622-1-55-B-5 Familie Lippmann.
[82]StAHH 352-3 IV C70 Wohlwill.
[83]StAHH 622-1-55-B-5 Familie Lippmann.
[84]Ibid.
[85]Ibid.
[86]Leo Baeck digital collection, papers of Richard Loewenberg. Letter from Friedrich Wohlwill, Hawthorne, Massachusetts, 17 June 1952 to Richard Loewenberg.
[87]Ibid.
[88]Ibid.

worked there instead from July 1953 until his death[89] (Andrae and van den Bussche, 1998). At Harvard, he conducted several research projects and published three papers on neuropathology of congenital early acquired encephalopathies, taught pathology to students and residents, lectured on the neurosciences and, since 1955, was consultant in the Cerebral Palsy Program with Yakovlev.[90]

In 1958, Wohlwill (and after his death his wife) tried to obtain the status of a full university professor in Germany, or at least get compensation for the fact he never was able to become one. This effort was aided by well-known scholars in German and American (neuro)pathology who testified to his expertise and wrote in confirmative letters that he would have become a full professor if had he not been forced to leave.[91] But Wohlwill's request was not granted because of negative advice from the Hamburg medical faculty. The well-known Jewish banker and philanthropist Eric Warburg (1900–1990) protested to the University Rector and even the Hamburg Ministry of Education but they were unwilling to overturn the position of the faculty. In June 1960, two and half years after the original request of Wohlwill, the Hamburg University administration and Wohlwill's widow compromised: Wohlwill was granted a lower wage category than that of a full professor together with an emeritus pension. The absurdity of this case becomes even more apparent considering that the same faculty had awarded Wohlwill the "Hermann-Kuemmel-Honorary-Medallion" on November 27, 1957 for "his great merits in science"[92]— two months before his application for promotion to full professor!

Richard D. L. Loewenberg

Richard D. L. Loewenberg (see Fig. 8) from Hamburg was the most junior of the five academics, and the earliest to flee the Reich. After obtaining his medical degree and completing internships, Loewenberg worked from 1927–1929 at the St. Georg neurological department. From 1929–1933, he was an assistant under Weygandt at Hamburg-

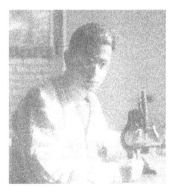

Figure 8. Richard Loewenberg using a microscope in Hamburg, 1930–1933. © Peter Loewenberg of Los Angeles, CA.

---

[89]Ibid.
[90]StAHH 352-3 IV C70 Wohlwill.
[91]StAHH 361-1 IV 1125 Wohlwill.
[92]Ibid.

Friedrichsberg, showing a particular interest in youth and social psychiatry.[93] Weygandt wrote a support letter for Loewenberg in 1933 praising his youth psychiatric care, his education of the nurses (see Fig. 9), and his care of "alcoholic maniacs," helping to found a *Guttemplerloge*.[94,95] Loewenberg also spent time working at the University Neurological Clinic under *Oberarzt* Georg Schaltenbrand (1897–1979), with Schaltenbrand in 1933 praising Loewenberg's work and stating that "he is obliged to quit his position here only because of the new legislation" (Loewenberg, 2012, p. 57).

Loewenberg was dismissed without pension as a "non-Aryan" in May 1933, effective by September 30.[96] This set off a worldwide involuntary odyssey for Loewenberg and his family eventually finding refuge in 1937 in California. With his wife being pregnant and realizing he had no future under the Nazis, Loewenberg initially visited the United Kingdom in May 1933 seeking help from the Joint Foreign Committee (an Anglo-Jewish Agency), the Jewish Refugees Committee, and Dr. Redcliffe Salaman (1874–1955). Salaman sent Loewenberg's papers, testimonials, and Curriculum Vitae to child psychiatrist Emanuel Miller (1892–1970) of the East London Child Guidance Clinic stating

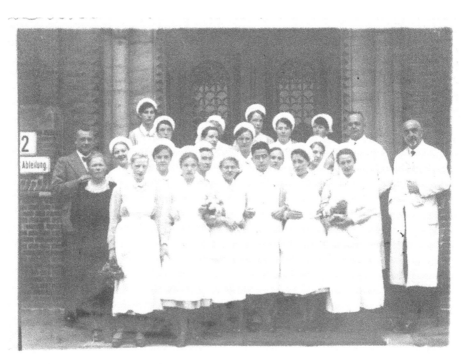

Figure 9. Richard Loewenberg in the center of a group of nurses who have just completed their training and examinations in Friedrichsberg, September 30, 1932. © Peter Loewenberg of Los Angeles, CA.

---

[93]StAHH, 351-11-27713, p. 195; Institut fuer Zeitgeschichte, Munich, Akte Loewenberg; Oxford Bodleian SPSL file 396-10: Loewenberg, Richard.
[94]The Good Templars are an international organization, currently called "IOGT International" (International Organization of Good Templars), dedicated to alcohol and illegal drug abstinence.
[95]Oxford Bodleian SPSL file 396-10: Loewenberg, Richard.
[96]Ibid.

that "he is clearly not one of the 'fliers' but I am wondering whether he seems to you of any use at all."[97] Miller was impressed by Loewenberg's credentials, but he did not think his publications revealed enough child or general psychiatric experience to "be of any use at our clinic, but he would certainly be a valuable member of a mental hospital staff."[98] Miller continued by stating the following:

> [C]ompetition for mental hospital jobs are very keen … [and] I doubt …whether a Home Office permit would be given to him as his work is not sufficiently unique to call for special consideration.[99]

After getting Miller's response, Salaman wrote, "I have tried again with Loewenberg, and unfortunately failed." The SPSL, Salaman, and Quastel were more successful in placing Josephy, as mentioned above, especially since Josephy only needed temporary unpaid positions.

Without viable options in Britain to obtain a British visa, Loewenberg investigated global options for escape, including Egypt, Aden, Tangiers, Persia, and even Ethiopia before settling on Shanghai (Loewenberg, 2012). Arriving in Shanghai in October 1933 with his wife and two-month-old baby, Loewenberg's reasons for choosing Shanghai were "No immigration restriction; Immediate practice of medicine."[100] Indeed, the internationally administered Free Zone of Shanghai had no visa requirement and was a transient safe haven for many refugee doctors who established medical practices there until they could re-emigrate (Kater, 1989b). Loewenberg's official application to the SPSL in February 1935 from Shanghai was as unfruitful as the earlier efforts he had made to find a position in the United Kingdom.[101] He stayed in Shanghai from 1933 to 1937,[102] maintaining a private psychiatric practice but also working as a consultant at the Polyclinic for Nervous Diseases of the Tung Nan Medical College, and was a member of the Medical Council of the International Settlement of Shanghai.[103] Loewenberg had expected to make Shanghai a permanent home, and his family integrated into the old established Jewish community there (Loewenberg, 2012). But the outbreak of the Sino-Japanese war in 1937 changed his plans, Loewenberg realizing he needed to immigrate again to the United States, which was "Distant, safe, free, [and there were] relatives there."[104] Loewenberg had learned English in Germany and used it in China, and his "family gave [an] affidavit of support for [a] visa."[105]

A distant cousin in El Paso, Texas, had sponsored Loewenberg's American visa, and he settled for several years in San Francisco. California medical licensing requirements required him to complete another rotating internship even at age 39. He spent a year working 120 hours a week and living in the hospital, earning only $25/month from 1937 to 1938 at St. Joseph's hospital in San Francisco, while his wife worked night shifts as a

---

[97]Ibid., p. 355.
[98]Ibid., p. 326.
[99]Ibid., p. 326.
[100]Institut fuer Zeitgeschichte, Muenchen, Akte Loewenberg.
[101]Oxford Bodleian SPSL file 396-10: Loewenberg, Richard.
[102]Institut fuer Zeitgeschichte, Muenchen, Akte Loewenberg; Leo Baeck collection, papers of Richard D. Loewenberg.
[103]Ibid.
[104]Institut fuer Zeitgeschichte, Muenchen, Akte Loewenberg.
[105]Ibid.

nurse (Loewenberg, 2012).[106] The schedule was so arduous that Loewenberg's young son Peter had to become a pediatrician's foster child in Berkeley for that year, Peter later stating "they weren't my family ... A lot of pain there" (Loewenberg, 2012, p. 59). Thereafter, with a California medical license in hand, Loewenberg worked on the St. Joseph staff as a psychiatrist and in private practice from 1938 to 1942 (Loewenberg, 2012).[107] From 1941 to 1942, like Josephy's internment in England, Loewenberg had "restricted movement as an enemy alien,"[108] despite fleeing Germany as a refugee and having already filed a naturalization petition in the United States in December 1937.[109] Loewenberg served the US War Procurement and Assignment Service from 1942–1944 as a railroad physician for Western Pacific Railroad's Hospital in Portola, California, and was naturalized as an American in 1943 (Loewenberg, 2012).[110] In 1945, he moved to Bakersfield, California,[111] according to his brother, " a place without a neuro-psychiatrist."[112] He maintained a private practice in psychiatry and was staff psychiatrist at Kern County General Hospital.[113] Loewenberg was the only psychiatrist in the county, while his liberal nurse wife (previously an anti-fascist and leftist in Germany) was active in the Jewish community but also in social justice causes, once helping young activist Cesar Chavez (1927–1993) to recover in their home after a hunger strike (Loewenberg, 2012). Loewenberg became a victim of McCarthyism: According to a private curriculum vitae written by a family member, "In 1948 he had to give up his well-paid position under the pressure of political medicine."[114] While delivering a lecture at the University of Southern California in Los Angeles, where he had become Clinical Professor of Psychiatry,[115] Loewenberg suffered a stroke and died tragically at age 56 (Loewenberg, 2012). After his death, his widow Sophie made a claim to the German *Amt fuer Wiedergutmachung*.[116] She finally accepted a settlement in 1961, far below her original claims.

"Making good again"?

The files of the Hamburg Medical Faculty show that no concerted effort was made after the war to renew contacts with those who had been expelled in 1933, despite the fact that the British Military Government had decided that these colleagues should be preferably considered for open positions in the whole British Zone (van den Bussche, 2014c). Kafka did return temporarily and was invited to lecture in 1949. Reasons for exiled faculty not returning were multiple. On both sides, everybody dedicated most energy to survival

---

[106]Ibid.
[107]Institut fuer Zeitgeschichte, Muenchen, Akte Loewenberg; Leo Baeck collection, papers of Richard Loewenberg.
[108]Institut fuer Zeitgeschichte, Muenchen, Akte Loewenberg.
[109]Petition for Naturalization 98809, Loewenberg, Richard. National Archives and Records Administration, Northern Division, San Bruno, California.
[110]Institut fuer Zeitgeschichte, Muenchen, Akte Loewenberg.
[111]Ibid.
[112]Leo Baeck collection, papers of Richard Loewenberg.
[113]Institut fuer Zeitgeschichte, Muenchen, Akte Loewenberg.
[114]Leo Baeck collection, papers of Richard D. Loewenberg (AR 6005), statement of family member of Loewenberg (Ernst?), undated.
[115]Institut fuer Zeitgeschichte, Muenchen, Akte Loewenberg.
[116]StAHH, 351-11, 27713.

matters (housing and food), many refugees had lost family members in the Holocaust and did not want anything to do with Germany, and many also heard about the disastrous living conditions in postwar Germany. On the other hand, faculty members were not eager to discuss how to handle the twofold filled positions (once by a Jew before 1933 and one by an "Aryan" afterwards), or their own complicity in "de-Jewification," and, last but not least, the spirit of the majority of the faculty members had not changed fundamentally because of the rapid return to office of the "denazified" (van den Bussche, 2014c). The most important preoccupation of the Nazis and non-Nazi "Aryan" beneficiaries was to secure their so-called political opposition and mere "inner emigration" during the Nazi era. In that sense, "*Persilscheine*," especially from Jewish former colleagues (Sachse, 2009), were an important tool.

"*Wiedergutmachung*," literally means "making good again" (Loewy, 1998) and could take place in financial or professional and academic terms. The academic reparation policy of the Hamburg faculty was usually in favor of the requesting exiled colleagues, but, as in Wohlwill's case, this was not always true. In the example of Kirschbaum, the faculty fully supported his reparation request but this may have been easier as the position in question was "only" an *Extraordinarius*, not a full professorship. In most cases, the victims obtained compensation after processes often lasting more than 10 years. By the late 1950s most material claims were resolved (Pross, 1998a).

Larger scale research and commemoration activities began only in the 1980s, somehow after the death of most persons immediately involved in Nazi activities. These activities concern single faculties and/or medical disciplines and their participation in Nazi programs, for example, compulsory sterilization and "euthanasia," especially for pediatrics and neurosciences. These activities are still unfinished and discussions continue in many places. As for the Hamburg Medical Faculty, research, teaching, and medical care for patients were extensively investigated during the 1980s and the biographies of all 16 dismissed professors reconstructed (van den Bussche, 1989). In his central speech at the one-hundredth anniversary of the founding of the university hospital in 1989, the Faculty Dean and Medical Director, in the presence of the only survivor of the expelled Jewish medical scientists, officially apologized for what had been done to the Jewish university physicians. The doctor titles withdrawn by the Nazis were finally reallocated in 1991 by the president and the Academic Senate of the university. The biographies of all exiled Jewish physicians from Hamburg were reconstructed with the support of the Hamburg Medical Association (von Villiez, 2009), which finally acknowledged its responsibility in 2005. At the one hundred twenty-fifth anniversary of the University Hospital in 2014, "stumbling stones" (*Stolpersteine*) were laid at the entrance of the hospital in commemoration of the 16 dismissed faculty members, among them the five neuroscientists described in this article (see Fig. 10). Discussions are ongoing, for example, regarding the persistence of the naming of the Leibniz-Institute for experimental virology as the "Heinrich Pette Institute" since 1948. The effects of *Gleichschaltung* still ripple through to the present day.

Discussion

Was it really "emigration" (Stahnisch, 2010) when these five neuroscientists were dismissed from hard-earned positions, legally robbed, intimidated and exiled from their

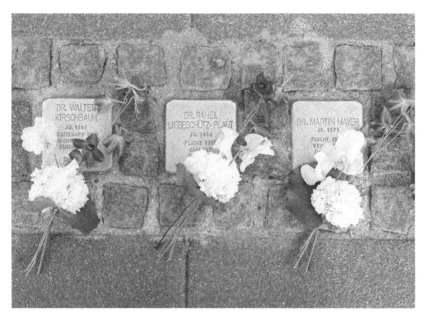

Figure 10. Walter R. Kirschbaum *stolperstein* installed in 2014 in front of the entrance of the University Hospital Hamburg-Eppendorf. There are also *stolpersteine* for Wohlwill, Josephy, and Kafka. © Hendrik van den Bussche of Hamburg, Germany.

fatherland for which some of them had fought during WWI? "Emigration" is a voluntary move from one country to another, not being disfranchised to the point where leaving, if possible, is the only viable option. Hamburg neuroscience was decapitated (Kater, 1989a) by the massive unjust and unethical removal of qualified personnel not just from a medical perspective but from the human and professional vacuum created by the ostracism and persecution of these individuals.

As all others, the five neuroscientists from Hamburg were victims of the racist Nazi politics. They lost their positions and titles, their workplace, and even medical instruments, such as Josephy's 580 RM microscope that had to be liquidated,[117] and lost most or all their private property. They fled for their lives (twice for Loewenberg and Kafka), three were imprisoned by the Nazis, and three were interned, detained, or restricted in movements as "enemy aliens" even after escape. They lost friends and family members in many cases, and all lost their culture and homeland. They received little help or support from their university, city, and country. Despite not protesting the injustice of dismissing Jewish colleagues, Nonne showed sympathy to Kafka, Wohlwill, and six other former trainees (Peiffer, 2004). Weygandt, an "Aryan" but forced into early retirement in 1934 because of outmaneuvering by a racial hygiene competitor (van den Bussche, 2014b), also supported Kirschbaum, Kafka, Loewenberg, and Josephy with letters of recommendation. Postwar there was never any outright apology by former Nazi colleagues, exemplified by Demme's inglorious memorial to Kafka. Some, like Kafka, Josephy, and Kirschbaum, waited many years before leaving Germany. All of them ended up, at least initially, in much less ideal conditions than those they had left. No one gained a rank of full professor abroad, a

---

[117]File from the "Devisenstelle" of the "Oberfinanzpraesident Hamburg", StAHH/OFP 314-15/F1204.

realistic perspective in their home country under democratic conditions. Abroad, some regained at best an academic position similar to the one lost in Hamburg, mostly after more than a decade. In the meantime, they had to work for a low salary, if paid at all. Resources for scientific research were almost absent, and they often had to work at least initially under more primitive clinical conditions than what they left in Hamburg. Like Wohlwill, Kirschbaum, and Josephy they had to take low-level research assistant positions and often had to live on hospital grounds or to work multiple simultaneous jobs to earn enough to feed their families. All this is in contrast to the theory that the Jewish emigrants played an important role in the scientific development of their host countries (Stahnisch, 2010). There have certainly been such cases, but a generalization in this respect rather seems like exculpation.

Overall trends of emigrant doctors from the German Reich are verified by these five representatives, in that 50% went to the United States, 22% to Palestine, 12% to the United Kingdom, 7% to other European countries (i.e., Sweden), and 1% to Asia (mainly Shanghai). Psychiatrists (including neurologists) made up the largest specialist portion of emigrant doctors (15%) and the largest proportion of immigrants to America (22.3%) (Kroener, 1989). These five neuroscientists overcame at least two large obstacles in that they were all under 60 and spoke some English. But on a more personal level, many emigration trajectories were significantly arduous. Loewenberg suffered from cultural and language difficulties in China as well as a lack of ability to build a thriving practice in neuropsychiatry. In Britain in the 1930s, refugee physicians were not allowed to practice medicine without studying again and repeating the final medical examination without a possibility to practice clinically (Kater, 1989b). Therefore, Britain became a transit station for most emigrants. British Palestine's borders were also closed to most medical immigrants especially in the late 1930s. Independently of the profession, changing visa quota and/or application deadlines prohibited a departure. Kirschbaum and Josephy faced the fact that the German quota for American visas was not filled at all until 1939 after *Kristallnacht* (Kater, 1989b). Josephy's MRH offer expired after his prolonged stay in England interned as an "enemy alien" and still waiting for a US visa. Also, neutral Sweden was not a popular option for immigrants: Border-crossers like Kafka were detained and obtained Swedish citizenship only many years after arrival (12 years for Kafka).

One major reason for the American preference was the distance from the war in Europe and the Pacific. Another reason was the relatively high proportion of positions available in the United States and the opportunity to reestablish one's medical career quickly, at least in those states with a liberal relicensing policy (Kohler, 1997), which was mostly due to a physician shortage as well as local attitudes. New York, Massachusetts, New Jersey, Connecticut, Maryland, and Illinois were the most liberal states for refugee physicians (Edsall, 1940), but 15 states relicensed refugee doctors (Kohler, 1997). These more liberal states did not require citizenship for licensure and fully recognized foreign medical degrees, which likely influenced Josephy and Kirschbaum in settling in Illinois, which was facing a physician shortage (Edsall & Putnam, 1941), especially for neuropsychiatrists in mental institutions. Illinois required a one-year long internship but had reserved MRH internship spots that Kirschbaum and Josephy utilized (Zeidman, 2014). Loewenberg also did not face strict relicensing requirements in California, but his gruelling internship requirement caused severe family difficulties.

Conclusions

These five expelled academic neuroscientists' lives were fractured and set on a trajectory on which they could not prioritize their careers. *Wiedergutmachung* implies more than mere restitution or reparations, but also healing and coming to terms with the past on both sides (Loewy, 1998). This should not only have been made for financial or academic losses to the victims but professional and psychological losses as well; in reality, psychic damage was not taken into account. German medical experts who were often previous collaborators in Nazi race hygiene measures ignored international study results on Nazi terror victim psychopathology and conducted examinations that often resulted in claim denials. The process itself resulted in a "retraumatization of persecutees" (Pross, 1998b). Even 30 years after German President Richard von Weizsaecker's (1920–2015) famous "the secret to reconciliation is remembering" speech (von Weizsaecker, 1985), although some apologies and commemorations have occurred, several medical faculties and scientific associations in Germany have never attempted to "make good again" with the victims.

Acknowledgments

We wish to thank Dr. Frank Stahnisch (Calgary) for inviting us to contribute to this special issue, Prof. Eckart Krause of the Universitaet Hamburg Arbeitsstelle und Bibliothek fuer Universitaetsgeschichte, the staff of the Hamburg Staatsarchiv, Stephen Wordsworth of the Council for At-Risk Academics (CARA, successor agency to the SPSL) for granting permission to research and reproduce AAC/SPSL files at Oxford, Colin Harris and the staff of the Oxford Bodleian Library (Weston Library, Oxford University, Oxford, England) for help with the AAC/SPSL files, the staff of the National Archives and Records Administration Great Lakes Division (Chicago, IL), Peter and Samuel Loewenberg (son and grandson of Richard Loewenberg, respectively), Jon Barstad (Norwegian Riksarkivet [Main State Archive], Oslo, Norway), Maynard Gerber (Cantor of The Great Synagogue in Stockholm, Sweden) for assistance with Kafka, Lars Hallberg (Swedish Riksarkivet Stockholm, Sweden), and Kristian Groenseth (Oslo, Norway) for help translating and interpreting Norwegian and Swedish files on Kafka.

Funding

Dr. Zeidman received support from the University of Illinois at Chicago Office of International Affairs (Nuveen International Development Fund).

References

Adelman GE (1987): *Encyclopedia of Neuroscience*. Basel, Birkhaeuser Verlag AG.

Andrae M, van den Bussche H (1998): Die Vertreibung der juedischen Aerzte des Krankenhauses St. Georg im Nationalsozialismus. *Hamburger Aerzteblatt* 52: 170–176.

Anonymous (1933, April): *Gesetz zur Wiederherstellung des Berufsbeamtentums vom 7*. Retrieved from http://www.documentarchiv.de/ns/beamtenges.html

Anonymous (1960, May 21): Obituary – Dr. Herman Josephy. *Chicago Daily Tribune*, p. 14.

Barkai A (2000): Juedisches Leben unter der Verfolgung. In: Meyer MA, ed., *Deutsch-Juedische Geschichte in der Neuzeit 1918–1945*. Muenchen, Verlag C. H. Beck, pp. 225–248.

Cohen MM (1997): The campaign against the Jews. In: *A Stand Against Tyranny: Norway's Physicians and the Nazis*. Detroit, Wayne State University Press, pp. 130–145.

Demme H (1930): Die Praktische und theoretische Bedeutung der Eiweissrelation im Liquor cerebrospinalis bei Nervenkrankheiten. *Archiv für Psychiatrie und Nervenkrankheiten* 92: 4–5.

Demme H (1951): Viktor Kafka zum 70. Geburtstag. *Der Nervenarzt* 22: 361.

Edsall DL (1940): The émigré physician in American medicine. *JAMA* 114: 1068–1073.

Edsall DL, Putnam TJ (1941): The émigré physician in America, 1941: A report of the national committee for resettlement of foreign physicians. *JAMA* 117: 1881–1888.

Holdorff B (2004): Founding years of clinical neurology in Berlin until 1933. *Journal of the History of the Neurosciences* 13: 223–238.

Janzen R (1977): Teaching neurology in Germany. *International Journal of Neurology* 11: 280–288.

Kafka V (1917): *Taschenbuch der praktischen Untersuchungsmethoden bei Nerven und Geisteskrankheiten.* Berlin, Verlag Julius Springer.

Kafka V (1930): *Die Zerebrospinalfluessigkeit.* Wien, F. Deuticke.

Kafka V, Kirschbaum WR (1922): Infektiöse nichtluetische Meningitis und Syphilis. *Deutsche Zeitschrift für Nervenheilkunde* 75: 1–3.

Kater MH (1989a): Medical faculties in crisis. In: *Doctors under Hitler.* Chapel Hill, University of North Carolina Press, pp. 111–149.

Kater MH (1989b): The persecution of Jewish physicians. In: *Doctors under Hitler.* Chapel Hill, University of North Carolina Press, pp. 177–221.

Kirschbaum WR (1968): *Jakob-Creutzfeldt Disease.* New York, American Elsevier Publishing Co.

Klee E (2005): *Das Personenlexikon zum Dritten Reich. Wer war was vor und nach 1945.* Frankfurt am Main, Fischer Taschenbuch Verlag.

Kohler ED (1997): *Relicensing Central European Refugee Physicians in the United States, 1933-1945.* Simon Wiesenthal Center Museum of Tolerance Online Multimedia Learning Center, Annual 6, Chapter 1. Retrieved from http://motlc.wiesenthal.com/site/pp.asp?c=gvKVLcMVIuG&b=395145

Kroener HP (1989): Die Emigration deutschsprachiger Mediziner im Nationalsozialismus. *Berichte zur Wissenschaftsgeschichte* 12 (Sonderheft): 1–44.

Kuller C (2004): Finanzverwaltung und Judenverfolgung. Antisemitische Fiskalpolitik und Verwaltungspraxis im Nationalsozialistischen Deutschland. *Zeitenblicke* 3(2). Retrieved from http://zeitenblicke.historicum.net/2004/02/kuller/index.html

Loewenberg S (2012): Loewenberg early history. In: Peter Loewenberg Festschrift. *Clio's Psyche* 19: 57–60.

Loewy EH (1998): Making good again, historical and ethical questions. In: Pross C, ed., *Paying for the Past: The Struggle over Reparations for Surviving Victims of the Nazi Terror.* Baltimore, Johns Hopkins Press, pp. 209–218.

Peiffer J (2004): *Hirnforschung in Deutschland 1849 bis 1974.* Berlin, Springer Verlag.

Pieper C (2003): Kurzbiographien. In: *Die Sozialstruktur der Chefärzte des Allgemeinen Krankenhauses Hamburg-Barmbek 1913 bis 1945: ein Beitrag zur kollektivbiographischen Forschung.* Münster, LIT Verlag, pp. 184–232.

Proctor RN (1988): Anti-semitism in the German medical community. In: *Racial Hygiene: Medicine Under the Nazis.* Cambridge, MA, Harvard Press, pp. 131–176.

Pross C (1998a): History. In: Pross C, ed., *Paying for the Past: The Struggle over Reparations for Surviving Victims of the Nazi Terror.* Baltimore, Johns Hopkins Press, pp. 19–70.

Pross C (1998b): Examiners and victims In: Pross C, ed., *Paying for the Past: The Struggle over Reparations for Surviving Victims of the Nazi Terror.* Baltimore, Johns Hopkins Press, pp. 106–164.

Sachse C (2009): "Whitewash Culture": How the Kaiser Wilhelm/Max Planck Society dealt with the Nazi past. In: Heim S, Sachse C, Walker W, eds., *The Kaiser Wilhelm Society under National Socialism.* Cambridge, Cambridge University Press, pp. 373–399.

Sammet K (2008): Alfons Jakob (1884–1931). *Journal of Neurology* 255: 1852–1853.

Schmuhl HW (2011): "Resources for each other": The society of German neurologists and psychiatrists and the Nazi "health leadership." *European Archives of Psychiatry and Clinical Neuroscience* 261: 197–201.

Shevell MI (1999): Neurosciences in the Third Reich: From ivory tower to death camps. *Canadian Journal of Neurological Science* 26: 132–138.

Stahnisch FW (2010): *German-Speaking Émigré Neuroscientists in North America after 1933: Critical Reflections on Emigration-Induced Scientific Change.* Preprint No. 403. Berlin, Max-Planck-Institut für Wissenschaftsgeschichte.

van den Bussche H (1989): *Medizinische Wissenschaft im "Dritten Reich." Kontinuität, Anpassung und Opposition an der Hamburger Medizinischen Fakultaet.* Berlin, Dietrich Reimer Verlag.

van den Bussche H (2014a): Die "Machtergreifung" an der Medizinischen Fakultaet. In: van den Bussche H, ed., *Die Hamburger Universitaetsmedizin im Nationalsozialismus.* Berlin, Dietrich Reimer Verlag, pp. 35–74.

van den Bussche H (2014b): Lehren und Lernen – Die aerztliche Ausbildung. In: van den Bussche H, ed., *Universitaetsmedizin Im Nationalsozialismus.* Berlin, Dietrich Reimer Verlag, pp. 275–340.

van den Bussche H (2014c): "Zusammenbruch" und Nachkriegszeit. In: van den Bussche H, ed., *Die Hamburger Universitaetsmedizin im Nationalsozialismus.* Berlin, Dietrich Reimer Verlag, pp. 397–427.

von Villiez A (2009): Biografien der Aerzte und Aerztinnen von A-Z (supplemental CD-ROM). In: Mit aller Kraft verdraengt, ed., *Entrechtung und Verfolgung "nicht arischer" Aerzte in Hamburg 1933 bis 1945.* Munich, Dölling und Galitz Verlag, pp. 1–115.

von Weizsaecker R (1985, May 8): *Speech to the German Bundestag, Bonn, May 8.* Retrieved from http://www.bundespraesident.de/SharedDocs/Reden/DE/Richard-von-Weizsaccker/Reden/1985/05/19850508_Rede.html

Zeidman LA (2014): *Neuroscientist Refugees from Nazi Germany Find Haven in Illinois.* Retrieved from http://www.hekint.org/index.php?option=com_content&view=article&id=1215

Zeidman LA, Kondziella D (2012): Neuroscience in Nazi Europe Part III: Victims of the Third Reich. *Canadian Journal of Neurological Sciences* 39: 729–746.

Between resentment and aid: German and Austrian psychiatrist and neurologist refugees in Great Britain since 1933

Aleksandra Loewenau

ABSTRACT
This article is a historiographical exploration of the experiences that German and Austrian émigré psychiatrists and neurologists made in Great Britain since 1933, after the Nazi Governments in Central Europe had ousted them from their positions. When placing these occurrences in a wider historiographical perspective, the in-depth analysis provided here also describes the living and working conditions of the refugee neuroscientists on the British Isles. In particular, it looks at the very elements and issues that influenced the international forced migration of physicians and psychiatrists during the 1930s and 1940s. Only a fraction of refugee neuroscientists had however been admitted to Britain. Those lucky ones were assisted by a number of charitable, local, and academic organizations. This article investigates the rather lethargic attitude of the British government and medical circles towards German-speaking Jewish refugee neuroscientists who wished to escape Nazi Germany. It will also analyze the help that those refugees received from the academic establishment and British Jewish organizations, while likewise examining the level and extent of the relationship between social and scientific resentments in Great Britain. A special consideration will be given to the aid programs that had already began in the first year after the Nazis had seized power in Germany, with the foundation of the British Assistance Council by Sir William Henry Beveridge (1879–1963) in 1933.

Introduction: Historical background

Signing the Versailles Treaty of 1919 was meant to guarantee peace in Europe; however, the political and economic situation on the continent was far from peaceful. The Weimar Republic, the successor of the defeated German Empire, struggled in fulfilling its obligations towards the Allies, including paying hefty war reparations (Schumann, 2012; McElligott, 2013). The loss of lucrative German territories, demilitarization of the Rhineland, and the limitation imposed on the armed forces (*Reichswehr*), in addition to pressure on Germany to take the sole responsibility for the war greatly affected the morale of its citizens and divided opinions among politicians (Schumann, 2012). The worldwide Great Depression of the late 1920s created a recession in the German economy and caused staggering unemployment. Moreover, reparation payments put the newly established republic on the edge of bankruptcy (Ritschl, 2013). The increasing dissatisfaction of the public with the government and the lack of political and financial stability contributed to German voters leaning towards the right-wing Nazi Party (NSDAP; The National Socialist German Worker's Party) led by Adolf Hitler (1889–1945) (Kolb, 2008). Moreover, the defeat of "White Russia" was a cause of greater concern amongst Europe's leaders; Bolshevism was viewed as a larger threat than Hitler's rise in Germany. This, and other factors played significant roles in the lack of a unified Western response to growing German aggression both at home and abroad. Hence, the Western Powers — Great Britain in particular — turned a blind eye to German violations of fundamental parts of the Versailles Treaty through its annexation of the Rhineland, Saarland, the unification (*Anschluss*) with Austria, and the invasion of the Sudetenland in the Czechoslovakia and the Memel regions (*Klaipėda*). Those expansionistic plans from the 1930s of the established "Third Reich" directly led to the outbreak of World War Two.

While the foreign-trade-dependent British economy struggled with the effects of the Great Depression in the early 1930s, the NSDAP had already claimed victory in the 1932 election, and a year later Hitler was proclaimed the Chancellor of the *Reich*. Soon, after the Nazis gained control over Germany, they attempted to eliminate all perceived enemies of their new state, such as socialists and communists (London, 2003, p. 25). Various laws were passed that focused on preserving the purity of the Aryan race. Early on, the Nazi racial policies and anti-Semitic propaganda targeted German Jews of every background from poor peasants to prominent scientists, lawyers, and representatives of the medical profession, among them were neurologists and psychiatrists who are one of the focuses of this article.

Three months after taking control over Germany, the Nazi government passed a new "Law on the Re-Establishment of a Professional Civil Service," according to which those with "non-Aryan decent" were forbidden from being employed in any branch of the civil service, and those already hired were dismissed (Longerich, 2010, p. 38). Contracts of thousands of tenured prominent academics were terminated. On April 22, 1933, the "The Decree on Admission of Physicians to Health Insurance Activity" was proclaimed. This effectively deprived a large number of Jewish physicians of their income (Sherman, 1973, p. 21). As result of additional regulations being passed between 1933 and 1938, Jewish physicians were allowed to practice their profession solely on other Jews (Majer, 2003).[1] Similar measures were applied to Jewish physicians in the annexed territories of Austria after the *Anschluss* (March 12, 1938) and Czechoslovakia, due to the Munich Agreement signed on September 29, 1938. Targeting Jewish physicians created a great shortage in public health care providers. According to British historian Paul Weindling's previous analysis, in 1933 in Berlin, there were 6,558 doctors, and 3,423 (52%) of them were classified by the Nazis as non-Aryans. Moreover, out of 4,900 doctors in Vienna in 1938, 3,200 were classified as Jewish under the Nuremberg laws (Weindling, 2010). Consequently, a number of Jewish physicians including prominent psychiatrists and neurologists began their efforts to escape the Nazi terror for Britain as early as 1933. After World War Two had broken out, most of those Jewish physicians who had remained

---

[1]See also the article by Zeidman, von Villiez, Stellmann, and van den Bussche (2016) in this special issue.

in the Third Reich were relocated to city ghettos and later transferred to the system of concentration and extermination camps, where most, with rare exceptions, perished.[2]

The attitude of the British government and medical organizations towards German-speaking refugee neurologists and psychiatrists

The first group of psychiatrists and neurologists who were forced to seek refuge in Great Britain during the early 1930s were German Jews. As emphasized in the introduction, German Jews were pushed out of their academic and practical positions due to governmental regulations based on race. Nazi interpretations of the mere term of a "Jewish person" were very vague and thus targeted those who practiced Judaism, had Jewish ancestors, Jews who converted to Protestantism or Catholicism, as well as gentile spouses that were married to Jews. Among the persecuted individuals were also gentile doctors who became dismissed because of their political beliefs or for openly disobeying Nazi rules. A large number of Jewish refugees — imagining the dark future of the Jewish population in Germany — were eager to leave their homeland as soon as the opportunity arose. During the early stage of the "Jewish crisis," between 1933 and 1934, Britain appeared as a rather unattractive destination to the majority of lay Jewish refugees, who preferred to relocate to the Netherlands or France, where many of them had relatives and friends in large urban Jewish communities. Furthermore, immigrating to Britain was costly, thus ordinary refugees preferred Palestine, the United States, and Latin or South America. Exceptions to this were those who were wealthy or held positions at universities or research institutes, for whom Britain was a country where they could further develop their academic careers (Niederland, 1991, p. 58).

By contrast, British Jews had themselves experienced various forms of discrimination during the Great Depression, due in large part to increasing support towards fascist ideologies in Great Britain as well, which reached its peak after the Nazis took control over Germany (Weindling, 2010, p. 246). Thus, immigration regulations — especially inspections of aliens upon arrival — were meticulously executed (London, 2003, p. 19). Potential immigration applicants to Great Britain faced various obstacles. One of them was a rather chaotic implementation of immigration policies. In 1933, Britain's Foreign Office still followed "The Aliens Order" (Cesarani, 1993, p. 38) passed in 1920, according to which only "rich and famous" aliens were desired and welcomed to settle on the British Isles. Effectively, this strict and selective policy also allowed admission of Jews who had business or family connections in Britain and highly skilled and internationally known professionals, including renowned academics, preferably Nobel prize winners (Moore, 1991, p. 70; Niederland, 1991, p. 60; Decker, 2003, p. 851). However, German physicians' credentials were not honored in Britain. Thus, in order to practice, they would have to go through often very long medical and professional relicensing processes.

The first groups of Jewish refugees from Nazi Germany arrived in Britain in January 1933. By the end of March, the number reached 400. At that point, the decision whether to admit someone or not was made by a government immigration officer upon arrival in

---

[2]One of the notable neurologists and psychiatrists who survived the concentration camps was the Austrian born Viktor Frankl (1905–1997) who was imprisoned at Theresienstadt, Auschwitz, and Dachau.

Britain. Generally, only temporary visitors were allowed to enter the country. Refugees were supposed to be dismissed. Although the number of newcomers at that point was not substantial, it was seen as a potential issue due to the financial implications it could entail on the British public, especially that a number of "visiting Jews" would had been unable to financially support themselves during a "supposedly short visit" (London, 2003, p. 27).

The attitude of the British medical circles towards alien psychiatrists and neurologists was in general quite resentful. The British Medical Association was known for their elite, conservative, and borderline chauvinistic approach not only towards alien doctors but also with respect to women, whose access to medical education was fairly limited, and their impact on British medicine practically nonexistent. The British Medical Association and the Medical Practitioners Union were not interested in introducing any changes — even if they would have improved the health care system (Weindling, 1991, p. 245, 2009). Although some physicians were in favor of employing foreign doctors, seeing them as potentially beneficial to the development of British medicine, the majority views and particularly those of the association board of both organizations could hardly be changed.

The opponents to such thinking claimed that the methods of continental schools of medicine was simply too different. British doctors viewed refugee practitioners — Germans, in particular — as threatening competitors in the medical marketplace (Weindling, 2007, p. 142). This attitude towards German refugee physicians was, for example, prominently expressed by the President of the Royal College of Physicians, Lord Dawson of Penn (1894–1945), who in November 1933, during discussions with the Home Secretary, stated that "the number that could usefully be absorbed or teach us anything could be counted on the fingers of one hand."[3] He additionally argued in favor of maintaining a strict entry policy and preventing alien students from seeking employment regardless of holding medical degrees obtained in Britain (Sherman, 1973, p. 49). More importantly, through its standardization of medical degrees that were awarded for research-based theses, German medicine was seen as a challenge that might lead to transformations of the medical education system in Britain (Weindling, 2007). Resentment was directed mainly towards medical practitioners rather than academics, as they were usually not expected to practice medicine alongside their research careers. Due to the social pressure of the medical establishment, the Home Office agreed to tighten the medical license regulations to further discourage foreign doctors from coming to Britain. Each newcomer soon had to take additional mandatory exams in anatomy and physiology, which delayed their employment. In Great Britain, each county self-regulated its medical license system, while in England the relicensing process took two years, in Scotland it took only one (Weindling, 1991, p. 248; Collins, 2009). Another option was clinical research, yet, in order to be admitted, refugee physicians needed to obtain a stipend and a research position.

The situation worsened after Austrian refugees began to arrive in larger numbers and the British Jewish association was no longer able to provide financial assistance for all. Thus, on May 21, 1938, despite great sympathy of the general public towards Austrian doctors, the British government introduced a visa entry system for all Germans and Austrians arriving after May 2nd "whether or not an applicant is likely to be an asset to the UK" (Sherman, 2013, p. 90; London, 2003, p. 63). Border officers were granted the

---

[3] The National Archives, Home Office 45/15882 Hoare, minute 23 November 1933.

right to grade and rank the refugees, and less desirable ordinary doctors — so called "rank and file" — could be refused entry (Moore, 1991, p. 72). The number of incoming immigration applications (200 per day) proved that the situation of Austrian Jews was continuously deteriorating. Some physicians who had other sponsors managed to enter the country as domestic servants. Negative opinion regarding the admittance of further groups of medical refugees was also expressed in the medical press. *The Lancet*, for example, published several reader letters in which medicine was presented as "an over-crowded profession" (Leys, 1938, p. 1182). This statement was "supported" by a too high number (187) — in the opinion of some of British MDs — of registered refugee medical practitioners. While some medical practitioners showed sympathy towards expelled scho-lars, the majority viewed them as competitors whose presence minimized the chances for future employment of local medical students or "decreased salaries" of the practicing British physicians (Leys, 1938, p. 1182). To some degree, the antagonism of the British public towards the newly arriving refugees was motivated by the Jewish origin of most of the German-speaking physicians in Britain (Honigsbaum, 1979, p. 276). Thus, as an alternative solution, it had been suggested that refugee physicians could be sent to the British colonies where there was a remarkable shortage of doctors (Hughes, 1938). In large numbers, however, British doctors resented working in the colonies due to the harsh tropical climate and undeveloped health care conditions.

While the Home Secretary, Sir Samuel Hoare (1880–1959), wished to bring 500 Austrian refugee physicians to Britain (Templewood, 1954), "The Medical Advisory Committee," under advice of the British Medical Association, rejected admitting Austrian physicians in large numbers. Instead, it postulated to limit the number of refugees to the bare minimum (a quota was established, which included 50 doctors from Austria and another 50 from Czechoslovakia). The committee further insisted on additional conditions to be met by all "newcomers," which included a completion of a compulsory two-yearlong clinical study prior to admission to practice following a detailed scrutiny of each applicant. In addition, Austrian doctors had no freedom of movement and were not allowed to settle in greater London, unlike German Jews who came to Britain between 1933 and 1936 (Sherman, 1973). According to contemporary press reports of the year 1938, the standpoint of the British Medical Association towards employment of medical refugees was too liberal and hence it "let down the 'little men' of the profession in agreeing to the admission of any alien doctors" (Shermann, 1973). This was, with minor exceptions, a general point of view among the British doctors. Not being able to obtain institutional or private assistance, some of the refugee physicians had to enter Britain as domestic servants — mainly women since it was easier for them to find a job or sponsor in a nonmedical area. A large number of physicians, however, worked on commission (per patient) or even pro bono in order to gain the relevant medical experience and to hope for a doctor's position in the British health care system later on.

The outbreak of World War Two later changed the prevailing attitude of the British government and the general public towards German-speaking refugees further. They were now seen as suspicious and as potential spies. British officials encouraged German-speak-ing refugees to return back to their home countries in 1939, but only 2,000 agreed to do so (Atkins, 2005, p. 61). Consequently, a large number of medical refugees were placed in internment camps, the most famous place of this internment process being Port Douglas on the Isle of Man between England and Northern Ireland.[4] The negative perception of the German-speaking refugees impacted their careers and many of them even lost their positions. Among those who were interned from the Maudsley Hospital in London, for example, had been the refugee neuroscientist Eric Guttmann (1896–1948), the Italian psychiatrist of Jewish origin, Amadeo Limentani (1913–1994), and a new neurology graduate, Felix Post (1913–2001) (Hilton, 2007, p. 218). Others detained were the following: the psychiatrist Herman Josephy (1896–1971) from the Runwell Hospital in Essex; the psychiatrist Erwin Stengel (1902–1973) of Bristol City Mental Hospital; and the neuro-pathologist Favel Friedrich Kino (b. 1882), who had fled to London from Frankfurt am Main in Germany.[5] Some of the detained refugee psychiatrists spoke very bitterly about their internment experience (see the personal Kino file in the collection of the Society for the Protection of Science and Learning).[6] Others proved their loyalty to the His Majesty King George VI (1895–1952) by joining the British forces, as did the refugee neurologist Eric D. Wittkower (1899–1983) (Leighton-Langer, 2006, p. 308).

The interment of German-speaking doctors during the period of worsening of the war led to a moderation of the government's attitude towards Medical Registration. In 1940, the Home Office Advisory Committee agreed that an employment of the refugees might be necessary; however, they demanded to prevent alien doctors from establishing "unauthorised private practice" (Weindling, 2007). In January 1941, the Temporary Registration Order was passed, which honored foreign qualifications and allowed the employment of alien doctors in the armed forces, preselected hospitals, and British-run private practices (Weindling, 2007, p. 149). The Emergency Medical Services were initially meant to recruit American doctors; however, it was much cheaper and more effective to employ physicians who were already living in Britain; Germans, Austrians, Poles, and Czechs were used for that purpose (Weindling, 1991, p. 247). Eventually, in 1942, the position of refugee neuroscientists improved visibly when the Ministry of Health introduced a plan to increase Britain's psychiatric health care resources (Roelcke, Weindling, & Westwood, 2010, p. 222). Within a decade, a majority of refugee psychiatrists and neurologists, who had remained in England, Wales, Scotland, and Northern Ireland, gained their qualification and later also British naturalization.

Help provided to refugees

The German crises and the increasingly troubled position of its Jewish population gathered considerable attention and sympathy from various groups among British and international societies. Within several months of Hitler's appointment, a number of relief and funding organizations had been established, which aimed to provide support to those escaping Germany and later the Nazi-occupied territories (see Table 1).

Most of the relief organizations were established in 1933, which suggests that the British population, particularly local Jewish communities, had a distinct awareness regarding the situation of Jews in Germany. As Table 1 presents, the number of Jewish organizations helping

---

[4]Other camps were located in Cotton Mill, Bertram Mills Circus, Devon Holliday Camp, and Press Heath. A number of refugees were later deported to camps in Canada and Australia in 1940.
[5]Bodleian Library, The Society for the Protection of Science and Learning (SPSL).
[6]Bodleian Library, SPSL Collection, File Favel Kino.

Table 1. Relief and funding organizations in Britain.[7]

Jewish Organizations	Gentile Organizations
• The Central British Fund for German Jewry (CBF) (1933) • Jewish Refugee Committee (JRC) (1933) later known as German Jewish Aid Committee (GJAC)* • Lord Baldwin Fund (1938) • Refugee Children's Movement (1936) • Council for German Jewry (1935) • Chief Rabbi's Religious Emergency Council • Joint Foreign Committee of the Board of Deputies and the Anglo-Jewish Association • Coordinating Committee for Refugees • General Advisory Council for Relief and Reconstruction (1933) • Women's Appeal Committee for German-Jewish Women and Children (1933) • Council for the Protection of Rights and interests of Jews form Germany (1945)	• Society of Friends' Germany Emergency Committee (later known as the Friends Committee for Refugee Aliens) (1933) • Bloomsbury House (1933) • Catholic Committee for Refugees from Germany *Academic Aid Organizations:* • Academic Assistance Council (AAC) renamed in 1936 as The Society for the Protection of Science and Learning (SPSL)** (1933) • The Rockefeller Foundation (RF) (although not a British organization the RF provided substantial funds for refugee scholars residing in Britain) (1933–1945) • International Students Services

*Abbreviation GJAC will be used throughout this article. **Abbreviation SPSL will be used throughout this article.

German-speaking refugees was quite diversified; nonetheless, gentile organizations — particularly those of them that represented academic aid committees — although focused on selected groups, provided a substantial help to medical as well as academic refugees.

Jewish organizations: German Jewish Aid Committee and Central British Fund

In 1933, a British baker and Prominent Jewish philanthropist, Otto Schiff (1875–1952), brought the "Jewish immigration issue" to the attention of the British Cabinet. Schiff had previously been involved in running an aid organization called the "Temporary Jewish Shelter," which was established in 1884 to help Jews fleeing the Russian pogroms (Sherman & Shatzkes, 2009). During several discussions with the British Home Office, Schiff guaranteed that any costs related to admitting Jewish refugees would be covered by the newly created Jewish Refugee Committee — later called the German Jewish Aid Committee (London, 2003, p. 26). Schiff's German Jewish Aid Committee aimed to provide "maintenance, training, employment, and re-migration" to German Jewish refugees (London, 2003). In exchange, Schiff was hoping that the government would relax entry requirements for Jews escaping Germany (Sherman, 1973, p. 260). From that point onwards, the German Jewish Aid Committee acted as the Jewish spokesman to the government and the Central British Fund for German Jewry focused on approaching wealthy Jews in Britain, mainly business owners, in order to secure necessary funds; both organizations worked in tandem. By acknowledging the Jewish crises in Germany through allowing refugees to enter the country and not making an official stand on that matter to avoid a political faux pas with Germany, the British government tried to maintain the "good trouble-free image" (London, 2003, p. 32). The Jewish community had estimated that the number of German refugees seeking asylum in Great Britain might reach 4,000.

---

[7]For the purpose of this article I will focus on achievements of the most prominent organizations, namely, GJAC, CBF, SPSL and the RF.

The British Cabinet, however, predicted that it would most definitely be much higher given that in early 1930s Germany's Jewish population was 500,000 (Sherman, 1973, p. 31). In order to minimize any potential tensions between refugees and the general public, the German Jewish Aid Committee instructed new Jewish refugees on respecting customs in Britain. Refugees were asked not to comment on religion and politics and to restrain from any criticism towards decisions that were made by the British government.[8] This, however, did not prevent the spread of negative attitudes towards the Jewish refugees.

After the *Anschluss* of Austria, the number of immigration applications increased dramatically. Soon after, the German Jewish Aid Committee announced that the number of new applications was overwhelming, and, therefore, they were no longer able to deal with the high demand necessary for financial support. As London points out, Schiff was unwilling to commit to the Austrian refugee issue. His support was offered only toward German Jews. The German Jewish Aid Committee likewise stood against admitting Jews from Czechoslovakia and from territories that had been threatened by Nazism like Poland and Italy (London, 2003, p. 129). Those in need for support continued receiving help from other Jewish and gentile institutions.

Academic help I: Academic Assistance Council — Society for the Protection of Science and Learning

In May 1933, a group of British academics led by the sociologist William Beveridge of the London School of Economics (LSE) established the Academic Assistance Council (AAC), later renamed the Society for the Protection of Sciences and Learning (SPSL), which aimed to provide financial help and temporary refuge to academics who "on grounds of their religion, race, or opinion were unable to continue to work in their own country" (Ruthenford, 1936, p. 607). Several British Nobel Prize winners supported Beveridge's initiative. Among them were the recipient of Nobel Prize in Physiology or Medicine in 1922, the physiologist Archibald Vivian Hill (1886–1977), and neuroscientist Charles Scott Sherrington (1857–1952), who was also awarded the Nobel Prize in Physiology or Medicine in 1932. Beveridge learned about the dismissal of German-Jewish academics during his trip to a conference in Vienna and was much appalled by the way the newly established German government treated its scientists. Beveridge's initiative soon received additional support from the Central Jewish Fund and, by August, the SPSL had raised close to £10,000. The SPSL used the money to provide one-year grants to academics in need. This help was meant to be only temporary as the SPSL and the Jewish community hoped that "Jewish crises in Germany" would end sooner or later. The SPSL offered two types of stipends: £250 per annum for scholars with families and £182 per annum for unmarried academics. The idea was to provide stipends and to assist in finding temporary placement for refugee academics at British universities and research institutes because this temporary employment was one of the requirements imposed by the British government (Zimmerman, 2006, p. 29).

---

[8]TNA, JML/1988.488, Brochure issued by the German Jewish Aid Committee http://webarchive.nationalarchives.gov.uk/±/http://www.movinghere.org.uk/deliveryfiles/JML/1988.488/0/1.pdf (Accessed on December 15, 2016).

By 1934, the Nazi racial policies had become ever more oppressive. It had become apparent that the crisis was no longer a temporary one and more extensive funds needed to be secured. The SPSL began to approach banks and other financial institutions, but the outcome was a rather marginal one. Another issue was finding permanent academic or medical placements for refugee professionals, which proved to be very difficult since hardly any British institution was able or willing to guarantee a placement. Moreover, anti-Semitism drove some refusals, yet most of the institutions struggled financially. Refugee scholars, in many cases, were allowed to use institutions' facilities free of charge. Despite such major obstacles since its inception, by 1937, the SPSL had supported 80 scholars in total from a wide range of disciplines, while continuing to support new ones as well. A year later, the number of permanently placed academics had increased to 127. The SPSL had also tried to partner with overseas organizations, primarily the Rockefeller Foundation (see the next section). Meanwhile, the SPSL changed its attitude towards the Jewish disenfranchisement through the genocide from politically restrained to more aggressive by openly condemning Nazi politics and oppression of scientists and physicians.

After the *Anschluss* of Austria, the crises deepened. A new approach had to be undertaken that aimed to find placement for the refugees at academic institutions and, in case of psychiatrists and neurologists, particularly in medical research departments. Overall, the SPSL provided help in gaining professional positions in Britain for at least 20 neuroscientists (see Table 2).

While analyzing the SPSL applications of the German-speaking neuroscientist, one can observe that, despite the age discrepancies, most of scholars came to Britain when they were between 28 and 41 years old. Among older scholars were Max Schacherl (60), Favel Kino (57), and Friedrich Lewy (54). Some mature German scholars, including Favel Kino,

Table 2. Neuroscientists helped by the SPSL.[9]

Name	Medical Specialization	Country of Origin*
Deutsch, Leopold	Psychiatry	Austria
Fleischhacker, Hans H.	Neurology	Germany
Herzberg, Alexander	Neurology	Germany
Jacoby, Ernst	Psychiatry	Germany
Josephy, Hermann	Neurology	Germany
Kahane, Robert	Psychiatry	Austria
Kino, Favel F.	Neuropathology	Germany
Klein, Robert	Neurology/Psychiatry	Czechoslovakia
Krapf, Edward	Psychiatry	Germany
Last, Samuel L.	Neurology/Psychiatry	Germany
Lewy, Friedrich H.	Neurology	Germany
Meyer, Alfred	Neuropathology	Germany
Pollak, Eugen	Neuropathology	Austria
Reitmann, Ferencz	Neurology	Hungary
Schacherl, Max	Neurology	Austria
Stengel, Erwin	Psychiatry	Austria
Stern, Karl	Psychiatry	Germany
Thorner, Hans A.	Neurology	Germany
Wittkower, Erich D.	Psychiatry	Germany
Zalud, Paul	Neurosurgeon	Czechoslovakia

*The country of origin is presented according to borders from 1930.

[9]Bodleian Library Oxford University; Collection: The Society for the Protection of Science and Learning (fond no. L. 20.11.).

Ernst Jacoby, and Hermann Josephy had to wait until 1939 to be admitted to Britain. Applications of younger neuroscientists, on the other hand, were processed more quickly, as most of them arrived in 1933 and in 1938 in the case of Austrian and Czech neuroscientists. Younger researchers, particularly those who were not married, were offered work in the tropical British colonies and, as was the case of psychiatrist Leopold Deutsch (b. 1896?), were willing to temporarily accept unpaid work.[10] Moreover, unlike in the case of the Rockefeller Foundation, older scholars experienced serious issues and delays awaiting their immigration. Max Schachrl's (1876–1964) application from 1938 was initially denied by the SPSL due to restrictions on the number of admitted Austrians. His file says that he came to Britain using his own financial resources. Schachrl was unable to find a paid job, even after the "Temporary Registration Order" had been enacted, which was attributed to his advanced age and poor knowledge of English.[11]

There has been a refined scholarly discussion between medical history research fellow Karola Decker, then at the Wellcome Institute, and Paul Weindling at Oxford Brookes University as to whether Britain was just a temporary destination for medical refugees (Decker, 2003; Weindling, 2009). Based on a deeper analysis of the historical materials in the SPSL collection, one could state that majority of neuroscientists, when asked about their preferred destination, put the United States on the top of their list. Some files are rather fragmentary; however, a minimum of 25% succeeded in obtaining posts in various North American institutions in addition to the neuropathologist Karl Stern (1906–1975)[12] and Erich Wittkower who eventually immigrated to Canada.[13] The fact that a relatively high number of psychiatrists and neurologists could remain in Britain can be explained by the relatively supportive attitude of the medical establishment and the British government towards this particular profession. Psychoanalyst refugees, to the contrary, — especially from the Viennese schools —became victims of intensified restrictive relicensing policies. Therefore, out of 120 psychoanalysts originally admitted to Britain only 14 remained, while the rest left, with a majority (80) immigrating to the United States (Ash, 1991, p. 103).

Academic help II: The Rockefeller Foundation

The Rockefeller Foundation had been engaged in supporting scientific research in Germany years before the Nazis had come to power. A major recipient of this funding was established in 1917: the German Research Institute for Psychiatry in Munich. Two important scholars, who created and ran the institute, were the psychiatrist Emil Kraepelin (1856–1926) and the epidemiologist and eugenicist Ernst Ruedin (1874–1952), who took over the institute's headship after Kraepelin's death in 1926. The German Research Institute for Psychiatry, as well as other research institutions, came under the influence of the new order imposed by Hitler. Thereafter, Ruedin supported the eugenics movement and compulsory sterilization of the mentally ill. While the German Research Institute for Psychiatry enjoyed some form of independence, it was partially funded by the

---

[10]Bodleian Library, SPSL Collection, File Leopold Deutsch.
[11]Bodleian Library, SPSL Collection, File Max Schechlr.
[12]See also the article by Stahnisch (2016) in this special issue.
[13]Bodleian Library, SPSL Collection.

government. Thus, the institute did not escape group dismissal of non-Aryan academics following the announcement of "the re-establishment of a professional civil service" (Cesarani, 1993, p. 39).[14] Moreover, Rockefeller fellows, most of whom were emerging scholars, were also nominated by their research institutions; thus, it was believed that their fate was in the hands of directors of those institutes. On some rare occasions, scholars who were recipients of long-term grants, were kept in place until completion of their grant, which was, for example, the case of the experimental biologist Viktor Hamburger (1900–2001) (Weindling, 2000, p. 480). In this manner, the German Research Institute for Psychiatry tried to maintain its worldwide reputation. The Rockefeller Foundation, on the other hand, did not wish to get involved in too many political complications, while hoping to maintain its apolitical stance.

Meanwhile, the onset of the Jewish academics' dismissals and consequently their exodus brought to the fore the issue of financial support, which the escaping scholars desperately needed to make a living in their new home countries. Many of those who chose to go to Britain began their efforts to gather supporting documents for their immigration applications. In 1933, the Rockefeller Foundation launched its "placement programme" that was addressed to help refugee scholars.[15] Struggling for funding, the SPSL approached the Rockefeller Foundation acting as something like a negotiator on behalf of refugees. The results were, however, less than optimistic. According to Rockefeller Foundation regulations, a potential recipient of an award had to be permanently employed at a research institution. In 1933/1934, this was quite impossible, as only a small number of refugees managed to obtain academic or research positions and all of these were meant to be temporary. In addition, candidates with stateless status were by rule disqualified. The Rockefeller Foundation was also not interested in becoming an official partner organization of the SPSL. After long negotiations, the Rockefeller Foundation finally agreed to support a limited number of neuroscientists (precisely 16) who received funding for up to three years in order to conduct research in Britain.[16] Among the individual recipients, however, were predominantly scholars with established positions who had already received Rockefeller Foundation funding in the past (Weindling, 2000, p. 481).

The requirements of the Rockefeller Foundation changed in 1940, after Hitler had invaded Scandinavia and France. The Rockefeller Foundation now acknowledged that at that point obtaining permanent positions in Europe was less probable for refugee academics, and a number of scholars were in danger of being imprisoned or even killed if they were to stay in Europe. Thus, in 1940, the Rockefeller Foundation announced a new Emergency Committee in Aid of Displaced Foreign Scholars in the United States, which it would financially support. The Rockefeller Foundation favored medical research and teaching, particularly in psychiatry, neurology, and psychology. The University of

---

[14]The "re-establishment of the professional civil service" applied mainly to publicly funded institutions, including universities, where approximately 20% of all scholars were dismissed.
[15]Rockefeller Foundation Report, 1940, according to which the RF allocated $ 775,000 on aid for refugee scholars of various disciplines. https://www.rockefellerfoundation.org/app/uploads/Annual-Report-1940.pdf (Accessed on 10 December).
[16]Approximately 20 medical refugees received financial support from the Rockefeller Foundation and many of them were employed at the Maudsley Hospital. Some were additionally supported by the SPSL, such as neuropathologist Alfred Mayer (1895–1990).

Edinburgh, for instance, received $18,250 for research on head injuries under the leadership of Professor David Kennedy Henderson (1884–1965) and Norman Dott (1897–1973). This was not the first support from the Rockefeller Foundation for the University of Edinburgh. In fact, most of the funding went to already existing projects, as was the case with the University of Oxford, which prior to 1940 had received $12,000 and in 1940 received an additional $2,409 for research into brain chemistry.[17] The funds were provided to selected institutions, which took part in the scheme, and most of the research grants were given for a minimum of one year. Individual applicants were not considered; thus, in order to receive the funds, refugee scholars had to obtain a position at those research institutions. This certainly proved to be quite difficult, particularly for junior scholars, due to the intensifying war and the successive decrease of funds for medical research.

Contributing to the science: German-speaking refugee psychiatrists and neurologists at Maudsley Hospital

Despite the various limitations that the British government had imposed on medical refugees, the position of neuroscientists — specifically clinical psychiatrists — was much better than that of other medical specialists. German psychiatry was seen as more advanced in research and clinical training, while German neuroscientists viewed mental illness as brain disease that needed to be diagnosed and treated in somatic terms. This theory had been invented and widely disseminated by the "German father of psychiatry" Emil Kraepelin (Shepherd, 2009, p. 462; Hayward, 2010, p. 68). In Britain, by that time, the mentally ill were often locked up in asylums without proper clinical treatment. In Germany, by contrast, psychiatry had developed rapidly since the late-nineteenth century and was regularly taught as a medical specialization at universities. Several large-scale psychiatric hospitals were established across the country, and psychiatrists were additionally trained in neurology and, unlike British trained psychiatrists, often had research and clinical experience (Weindling, 1991, p. 245; Shepherd, 2009, p. 461). Thus, when "the Jewish crises" erupted in Germany, the more progressive psychiatric institutions in Britain, such as the Maudsley that effectively operated on Kraepelin's model and the Bethlem Royal Hospital, being monetary supported by the London County Council, the Rockefeller Foundation, the Medical Research Council, and the SPSL joined their efforts to bring prominent German scholars to Britain (Jones, Rahman & Woolven, 2007, p. 357). Several renowned German scholars were brought in, among them were the following: neuropathologist Alfred Mayer, who was regarded as a mentor by many British

---

[17]Prior to 1940, the Medical Research Council in London received $42,968 for research in endocrinology, psychiatry, neurology, and allied subjects (in 1940, it received $4,574.77); research in hereditary mental diseases prior to 1940 received $9,235.26 (in 1940, the amount was $2,510.27); the Royal Medico-Psychological Association of London prior to 1940 received $4,715 and in 1940 received $3,216.57 for teaching and training in psychiatry. The Travistock Clinic in London prior to 1940 received $17,859.38 and, in 1940, received $2,433.14 for research on psychosomatic medicine. The Maudsley Hospital prior to 1940 received $103,681.25 and, in 1940, was awarded an additional $26,257.13. The Rockefeller Foundation Report, 1940. https://www.rockefellerfoundation.org/app/uploads/Annual-Report-1940.pdf (accessed on December 10, 2015).

psychiatrists and who escaped Germany with the help of SPSL; Willi Mayer-Gross (1889–1961) from Heidelberg University arrived in Britain in 1933; University of Bonn's neuro-pathology professor Erich Wittkower was also helped by SPSL and arrived in Britain 1933, where he investigated respiratory abnormalities in schizophrenia; as well as neurologist Eric Guttmann from Breslau, who was supported by the Rockefeller Foundation (Jones, 2009). In addition, there was a demand for specialists in psychotherapy, many of whom were Viennese Austrians who, thanks to their advanced and innovative techniques, found positions at Maudsley. Altogether 11 refugee neuroscientists found new employment at Maudsley (Hilton, 2007, p. 210; Shepherd, 2009, p. 463; Hayward, 2010, p. 78). According to London historian of psychiatry Claire Hilton's observation, Maudsley was unique in the respect that this hospital and research center employed a relatively high proportion of German-speaking refugee doctors, which could be explained by the fact that neuroscience was rather undeveloped in Britain and not particularly desired among the existing medicine specializations; therefore, it was easier to get a post as a psychiatrist rather than a surgeon (Hilton, 2007, pp. 215 and 222).

Conclusion

Refugee psychiatrists, who had trained at the more research-minded German-speaking universities, were more easily accommodated in the British health care system than many other medical specialists. This statement is supported by the fact that psychiatry was rather undeveloped in Britain and particularly refugee neuroscientists were viewed as assets and not primarily as competitors to their British colleagues. Refugee specialists in prestigious specializations, such as internal medicine or surgery, often struggled with the limitations that were imposed by the British government, as well as the reluctance of the medical establishment and the general public's distrust (Shepherd, 2009, p. 467). However, the stress related to immigration, the resentment of the British medical establishment, limited opportunities, and restrictions imposed on refugees caused a large number of medical refugees to treat Britain as a temporary refuge as they awaited their move to the United States. Constant bombing by the German *Luftwaffe* in 1940 created an atmosphere of uncertainty, while the refugees were themselves afraid that Britain might be invaded, so a majority of them tried to leave before the end of the war. Sadly, a number of them could not cope with the trauma and took their own lives, among them was Wilhelm Stekel (1868–1940) from the Bukovina, who had received his graduate medical and psychiatry training at the Vienna Medical School (Roelcke, Weindling, & Westwood, 2010, pp. 221 and 224).

Due to the Nazi racial discriminations, between 500,000 and 600,000 Jews applied to immigrate to Great Britain, while only 1 in 10 of them had been successful. New admissions of refugee medical practitioners were constantly vetoed by the British medical establishment (London, 2003, p. 131). Yet, the situation of medical researchers and clinicians was equally hard despite the financial help from the SPSL and the Rockefeller Foundation. It remains to be determined, in future historical research, how the work of the neuroscientists who remained in Britain was later received after the war. Likewise, the particular preference of the refugee psychiatrists and neurologists who tried to immigrate to the United States should also be further determined. Various historians, such as David Zimmerman from the University of Victoria in Canada, have described the activity of the

SPSL as an organization that was driven by political and scientific considerations. It will, therefore, be important to investigate the specific review and decision-making processes that went into the individual application files and how the neuroscientists compared to any other medical, surgery, and public health groups supported by this important aid organization. This could be a potential area for further research.

Acknowledgments

The author would like to express her sincere gratitude to Dr. Frank Stahnisch and Prof. Paul Weindling for their advice and assistance in writing this article.

Funding

The author acknowledges support for this study through an open operating grant (PI: Dr. Frank W. Stahnisch, University of Calgary) by the Canadian Institutes for Health Research (No/EOG-123690), as well as postdoctoral fellowship support by the Calgary Institute for the Humanities, University of Calgary, Alberta, Canada.

References

Ash M (1991): Central European émigré psychologists and psychoanalysts in the United Kingdom. In: Carlebach J, Hirschfeld G, Newman A, Paucker A, eds., *Second Chance: Two Centuries of German-Speaking Jews in the United Kingdom*. Tuebingen, J. C. B. Mohr, pp. 101–121.

Atkins EA (2005): "You must all be interned": Identity among internees in Great Britain during World War II. *The Gettysburg Historical Journal* 4: 59–92.

Cesarani D (1993): An alien concept? The continuity of anti-alienist in British society before 1945. In: Cesarani D, Kushner T, eds., *The Internment of Aliens in Twentieth Century Britain*. London, Frank Cass, pp. 25–52.

Collins K (2009): European refugee physicians in Scotland, 1933–1945. *Social History of Medicine* 22: 513–530.

Decker K (2003): Divisions and diversity: The complexities of medical refuge in Britain, 1933–1948. *Bulletin of the History of Medicine* 77: 850–873.

Hayward R (2010): Germany and the making of English psychiatry: The Maudsley Hospital 1908–1939. In: Roelcke V, Weindling P, Westwood L, eds., *International Relations in Psychiatry: Britain, Germany, and the United States to World War II*. Rochester, University of Rochester Press, pp. 67–90..

Hilton C (2007): A Jewish contribution to British psychiatry: Edward Mapother, Aubrey Lewis and their Jewish and refugee colleagues at the Bethlem and Maudsley Hospital. *Jewish Historical Studies* 41: 209–229.

Honigsbaum F (1979): *The Division in British Medicine: A History of the Separation of General Practice from Hospital Care, 1911–1968*. London, Kagan Page.

Hughes H (1938): An overcrowded Profession? *Lancet* 231: 1135.

Jones E (2009): The Maudsley Hospital and the Rockefeller Foundation: The impact of philanthropy on research and training. *Medical History* 64: 273–299.

Jones E, Rahman S, Woolven R (2007): The Maudsley Hospital: Design and strategic direction, 1923–1939. *Medical History* 51: 357–378.

Kolb E (2008): *The Weimar Republic*. London and New York, Routledge.

Leighton-Langer P (2006): *The King's Own Loyal Enemy Aliens: German and Austrian Refugees in Britain's Armed Forces, 1939–45*. Elstree,Vallentine Mitchell.

Leys D (1938): An overcrowded profession? *The Lancet* 231: 1182–1183.

London L (2003): *Whitehall and the Jews, 1933–1948: British Immigration Policy, Jewish Refugees and the Holocaust.* Cambridge, Cambridge University Press.

Longerich P (2010): *Holocaust: The Nazi Persecution and Murder of the Jews.* Oxford, Oxford University Press.

Majer D (2003): *Non-Germans Under the Third Reich: The Nazi Judicial and Administrative System in Germany and Occupied Eastern Europe with Special Regad to Occupied Poland, 1939–1945.* Washington, DC, United States, Holocaut Memorian Museum.

McElligott A (2013): *Rethinking the Weimar Republic: Authority and Authoritarianism, 1916–1936.* London, Bloomsbury.

Moore B (1991): Areas of reception in the United Kingdom: 1933–1945. In: Carlebach J, Hirschfeld G, Newman A, Paucker A, eds., *Second Chance: Two Centuries of German-Speaking Jews in the United Kingdom.* Tuebingen, J. C. B. Mohr, pp. 69–81.

Niederland D (1991): Areas of departure from Nazi Germany and the social structure of the emigrants. In: Carlebach J, Hirschfeld G, Newman A, Paucker A, eds., *Second Chance: Two Centuries of German-Speaking Jews in the United Kingdom.* Tuebingen, J. C. B. Mohr, pp. 57–68.

Ritschl A (2013): Reparations, deficits, and debt default: The Great Depression in Germany. In: Crafts N, Fearon P, eds., *The Great Depression of the 1930s: Lessons for Today.* Oxford, Oxford Press, pp. 110–139.

Roelcke V, Weindling P, Westwood L (2010): *International Relations in Psychiatry: Britain, Germany, and the United States to World War II.* Rochester, University of Rochester Press.

Rutherford E (1936): The society for the protection of science and learning. *British Medical Journal* 1(3924): 607.

Schumann D (2012): *Political Violence in the Weimar Republic, 1918–1933: Fight for the Streets and Fear of Civil War.* New York and Oxford, Berghahn Books.

Shepherd M (2009): The impact of Germanic refugees on twentieth-century British Psychiatry. *Social History of Medicine* 22: 461–469.

Sherman A (1973): *Island Refuge: Britain and Refugees from the Third Reich 1933–1939.* Ilford, Frank Cass & Co.

Sherman AJ, Shatzkes P (2009): Otto M. Schiff (1875–1952), unsung rescuer. *The Leo Baeck Institute Yearbook* 54: 243–271.

Stahnisch FW (2016): Learning soft skills the hard way: Historiographical considerations on the cultural adjustment process of German-speaking émigré neuroscientists in Canada, 1933 to 1963. *Journal of the History of the Neurosciences* 25: 299–319.

Templewood S (1954): *Nine Troubled Years.* London, Greenwood Press.

Weindling P (1991): The contribution of central European Jews to medical science and practice in Britian, the 1930s to 1950s. In: Carlebach J, Hirschfeld G, Newman A, Paucker A, eds., *Second Chance: Two Centuries of German-Speaking Jews in the United Kingdom.* Tuebingen, J. C. B. Mohr, pp. 243–255.

Weindling P (2000): An overloaded ark?: The Rockefeller Foundation and refugee medical scientists, 1933–45. *Studies in History and Philosophy of Biological and Biomedical Sciences* 31: 477–489.

Weindling P (2007): Medical refugees as practitioners and patients: Public, private and practice records. In: Hammel A, Grenville A, eds., *Yearbook of the Research Centre for German and Austrian Exile Studies.* Amsterdam, Editions Rodopi, pp. 141–154.

Weindling P (2009) Medical refugees and the modernisation of British medicine, 1930–1960. *Social History of Medicine* 3: 489–519.

Weindling P (2010): Alien psychiatrists: The British assimilation of psychiatric refugees, 1930–1950. In: Roelcke V, Weindling P, Westwood L, eds., *International Relations in Psychiatry: Britain, Germany, and the United States to World War II.* Rochester, University of Rochester Press, pp. 218–236.

Zeidman LA, von Villiez A, Stellmann J-P, van den Bussche H (2016): "History had taken such a large piece out of my life" — Neuroscientist refugees from Hamburg during National Socialism. *Journal of the History of the Neurosciences* 25: 275–298.

Zimmerman D (2006): The Society for the Protection of Science and Learning and the politicization of British science in the 1930s. *Minerva* 44: 22–45.

Emigrated neuroscientists from Berlin to North America

Bernd Holdorff

ABSTRACT

The highest number of German scholars and physicians, forced by the National Socialist regime to emigrate for "race" or political reasons, were from Berlin. Language and medical exams were requested differently in their new host country—the United States—leading to a concentration of immigrants in the New York and Boston areas. Very early Emergency Committees in Aid of German Scholars and Physicians were established. Undergraduate students (like F. A. Freyhan, H. Lehmann, and H.-L. Teuber) from Berlin seemed to integrate easily, in contrast to colleagues of more advanced age. Some of the former chiefs and senior assistants of Berlin's neurological departments could achieve a successful resettlement (C. E. Benda, E. Haase, C. F. List, and F. Quadfasel) and some a minor degree of success (F. H. Lewy and K. Goldstein). A group of neuropsychiatrists from Bonhoeffer's staff at the Berlin Charité Hospital could rely on the forceful intercession of their former chief. The impact of the émigré colleagues on North American neuroscience is traced in some cases. Apart from the influential field of psychoanalysis, a more diffuse infiltration of German and European neuropsychiatry may be assumed. The contribution to the postwar blossoming of neuropsychology by the émigré neuroscientists K. Goldstein, F. Quadfasel, and H.-L. Teuber is demonstrated in this article.

This article focuses on the settlement of emigrating German-speaking neuropsychiatrists and neuroscientists from the wider Berlin area to the United States. The main emphasis will be put on the movement of "brain gain" in America *vis-à-vis* the "brain drain" in Germany; that is, the question if a second career and a measurable impact on North American neuroscience could be identified. It is beyond the scope of this survey to detail the full working biographies of these colleagues in clinical neurological clinics prior to their immigration, as well as their importance for German neurology and neuropathology, which has been described elsewhere (Peiffer, 1998). Their working context in Berlin has been described in particular by Holdorff (2004) for the clinical neurology field.

Professional conditions of medical émigrés in the United States

The forced migration of Jewish physicians in Germany was initiated through the inauguration of the Nazi "Law on the Re-Establishment of the Professional Civil

Service" (*Gesetz zur Wiederherstellung des Berufsbeamtentums*) from April 7, 1933.[1] During the same year, when the first refugees reached their new host countries, primarily in the United States, various medical and social assistance groups had also come into existence. However, in 1933, the American Medical Association (AMA) was one of the largest and most powerful pressure groups for the protection of medical interests in the United States became engaged in a campaign to restrict the relicensing for foreign-educated physicians in the United States (Pearle, 1981, p. 14). More than half of the American states made official citizenship in the United States an obligatory requirement for the medical relicensing process, while most of them also required a professional exam before allowing foreign physicians to resume their medical practice. The states of New York and Massachusetts however had some of the most liberal licensing laws, initially requiring only a language test. They conferred a foreign medical license by professional endorsement until October 15, 1936 when medical exams were made mandatory for all immigrants. Four of the émigré candidates went to court after they had failed the examination and eventually succeeded in having their case vindicated (Pearle, 1981, pp. 47–184). Another famous petitioner, however, Prof. Dr. Otto Marburg (1874–1948), the former chair of the Institute of Neurology at the University of Vienna, who wanted to be reconsidered for medical practice, lost his lawsuit in July 1941 (Pearle, 1981, p. 225).

On the one hand, the hostile attitude towards refugee doctors by the professional medical community could be explained by several factors: the economic fear of an overcrowding of the profession, the nation was still suffering from the Great Depression during the first years of the 1930s (Kater, 1989, p. 210), xenophobia (Rypin, 1937, as cited by Pearle, 1981), and anti-Semitism among the membership groups of the AMA (Kroener, 1988) as well as in the US medical education system (Halperin, 1955, as cited by Zeidman & Kondziella, 2012). On the other hand, solidarity of the American society largely prevailed. Some private aid foundations had, for example, been founded only months after the "Law on the Re-Establishment of the Professional Civil Service" had come into effect in Nazi Germany (Pearle 1981, p. 29, 39). In June 1933, the "Emergency Committee in Aid of Displaced German Scholars" was founded, later called "Emergency Committee in Aid of Displaced Foreign Scholars." It had three guiding principles (Duggan 1941): (1) To support only institutions, not individual scholars, and preference to Americans in cases of equal merit, (2) to spend grants only to mature scholars between 30 and 58 years of age; and (3) to expect that the scholar be absorbed by the institution in its faculty (resulting in a success rate of about half of the cases). Mostly, these grants were duplicated by the Rockefeller Foundation to the sum of $2,000 per year (Duggan, 1941).

In October 1933, Bernard Sachs (1858–1944), who was the acting president of the New York Academy of Medicine (NYAM) and who was familiar with European medicine through his own postgraduate neurological training, cofounded a specialized Committee in Aid of Displaced Physicians. Between 1933 and 1942, it evolved into the most reliable relief organization for the resettlement of the newly arriving émigrés in America (Pearle, 1981, pp. 210–217).

---

[1] Reichsgesetzesblatt (statute for the restoration of the civil service) 1933, I, pp. 175–177; further reading: Fijal (1994).

The majority of the foreign physicians were not scientists and scholars and yet can be seen as belonging to the group of practicing physicians; their impact on U.S. medicine, however, can only hardly be assessed or even quantified. Their medical education level prior to their forced migration differed markedly to the North American one, both in terms of content variances as well as language problems. The acute shortage of doctors during WWII seemed to greatly improve the refugee physicians' chances of integration into American society (Pearle, 1981, p. 30). Nevertheless, xenophobic attitudes and antirefugee resentments had to be noted as well, at a time when medical boards did not accept Jewish members and when numerus clausa (NCs) existed at many American medical schools for students of Jewish faith (Kater, 1989, p. 211).

The list of displaced German scholars until 1936/1937 (Strauss et al., 1987, pp. 69–73, suppl. p. 10) contains 62 mostly Jewish scholars in clinical neurology, psychiatry, psychopathology, and psychotherapy. The majority were neuropsychiatrists, not neurologists, due to the German tradition of combining both specialties in education and practice (see also Stahnisch, 2008, pp. 443–446). The high percentage of immigrating neuropsychiatrists, the largest group of medical specialists following to that of the internists, is striking in this regard: They represented the classical nerve doctors (*Nervenaerzte*) in the tradition of Emil Kraepelin (1856–1926) in Munich and Julius Wagner-Jauregg (1857–1940) in Vienna (Kroener, 1988, pp. 2573–2578), while others stood for psychoanalytically oriented or dynamic psychiatry (Peters, 1992, 2008), including the different psychoanalytical schools. Most of the émigré neuropsychiatrists could not fully re-establish their former professional quality, not at least due to their initial or enduring language problems. Several neuropsychiatrists continued practicing but failed the licensing exam. Some young students from Berlin, among those forced to emigrate to North America, seemed to have had the best chances for a successful acculturation in their new homeland.

Medical students from the University of Berlin

The following students and trainees only later qualified as clinical or basic neuroscientists during their career in the United States:

Hans-Lukas Teuber

Hans-Lukas Teuber (1916–1977) had received a classical education at the French Gymnasium College in Berlin and studied biology and philosophy at the University of Basel in Switzerland. In 1941, Teuber came to the Department of Psychology at Harvard University as a graduate student and, in the same year, married Marianne Liepe an art historian. She came to play a central role in the groups (sometimes referred to as extended families) that later formed his experimental psychology laboratory at New York University, as well as the groups in his department at the Massachusetts Institute of Technology (MIT) in Cambridge, Massachusetts. Teuber's most important educational experiences during his graduate school period were probably the two years that he had spent away from his studies in the US Navy. During this time, he began to work with the neurologist Morris B. Bender (1905–1983) at the San Diego Naval Hospital on the effects of human brain lesions in injured soldiers. This collaboration lasted more than 15 years and produced a series of important neuropsychological articles, particularly on the effects of penetrating head wounds vis-à-vis visual and haptic functioning (Teuber, 1960). After returning to Cambridge, Teuber completed his doctoral dissertation at Harvard in 1947, which was based on a study of the effects of psychotherapy on teenagers with risk for delinquency. In 1947, Teuber established his Psychophysiological Laboratory at the New York University's Bellevue Medical Center.

A systematic experimental neuropsychology program had been pioneered and established at Bellevue, which led to a transformation of the study of human brain function from collected data of single neurological case reports. Teuber joined the Massachusetts Institute of Technology in the fall of 1961, where he was hired to organize a new department of psychology. Over the next decade, this became a world center for the behaviorally oriented neurosciences. He also ventured to study the case of H. M. in Canada. This epilepsy surgery patient had memory deficits after bilateral removal of the temporal hemispheric poles of his brain. Teuber applied new standards in neuropsychology and delivered revisions of the classical, anatomically based distinction between perception and cognition (Teuber, 1960). It transcended classical views of perceptual neurological disorders such as visual object agnosia (Teuber, 1965; Milner & Teuber, 1968), simultaneous agnosia, and other conditions. Teuber was a prolific scientific author (Teuber, 1978), who was also highly esteemed by European neuropsychologists such as Henri Hécaen (1912–1983; Hécaen, 1979) in France or Klaus Poeck (1926-2006; Poeck, 1982) in Germany, and Teuber was also a charismatic teacher at every level of undergraduate and postgraduate education in psychology and neurology (Hurvich, Jameson, & Rosenblith, 1987).

Fritz A. Freyhan

Dr. Fritz A. Freyhan (1912–1982) was born in Berlin and came to the United States in 1937 after graduating from the University of Berlin. His research in the 1950s examined the use of drugs for the treatment of psychosis and depression. He had interned at Sydenham Hospital in New York and then joined the staff of Delaware State Hospital, in Wilmington, in 1940. In 1961, he went to the National Institute of Mental Health in Bethesda, Maryland, where he worked for five years before he was appointed director of research at St. Vincent's. Five years later, he became the research director at St. Vincent's Hospital and Medical Center in Manhattan, New York City. Several papers and books dealing with social psychiatry or psychiatric care attest to his engagement in modern psychiatry. In 1972, Freyhan retired and went into private practice in Washington, DC.

Heinz Lehmann

Heinz Lehmann (1911–1999) received his MD at the University of Berlin in 1935 at a young age and was then forced to migrate to Montreal, Canada, where — as an untrained psychiatrist — he initially conducted ethically dubious therapies in psychiatric patients and later introduced chlorpromazine to North America in 1953 (Shorter, 1997, pp. 248–251). He eventually became one of the most prominent champions of modern psychopharmacology as the chair of the McGill University Department of Psychiatry at the Allan Memorial Institute (Stahnisch, 2008).

Bonhoeffer's coworkers

Karl Bonhoeffer

Karl Bonhoeffer (1868–1948), Director of the Neuropsychiatric Clinic (*Psychiatrische und Nervenklinik*) at the Charité Hospital in Berlin from 1912 to 1938, played an important role in delaying the dismissal of his Jewish coworkers and supporting their emigration to secure foreign countries — most of them leaving for the United States (see Table 1). Two physicians, Edith Jacobson (1897–1978) and Alfred Quadfasel (1902–1970), were even imprisoned by the Nazi regime for political accusations, for two years and two months, before being allowed to leave the country. Bonhoeffer delayed the dismissal of his most experienced coworker, Prof. Dr. med. Franz Kramer (1878–1967), until 1935. Kramer settled down in a private practice by 1938 and immigrated thereafter to the Netherlands where his medical prospects were poor during the Nazi occupation and at times he had to work as a physician in secret locations.

Hans Pollnow

Kramer's colleague, Dr. med., Dr. phil. Hans Pollnow (1902–1943) had been his coauthor on scientific papers on hyperkinesia in children (Kramer & Pollnow, 1930, 1932; for the Kramer-Pollnow-Syndrome, see Neumaerker, 2005). Pollnow fled to France, where he was caught by the Nazi persecutors (Gestapo) and eventually murdered in the concentration camp Mauthausen in Austria on October 21, 1943.

Hanns Schwarz

At the turn of 1938/1939, Dr. Hanns Schwarz (1898–1977) attempted to settle down in the United States but, disappointed about the materialistic competition among the physicians and the language problems of a foreign psychiatrist, he soon returned to. And thereafter,

Table 1. Coworkers of Karl Bonhoeffer, who were forced to emigrate to the United States.

Name	Main Research Subject	First Exile	Final Exile
Seidemann, Herta (1900–1984)	Dyslexia (prepared for habilitation thesis)	Switzerland, 1933 to 1936	New York, 1937
Jacobson, Edith (1897–1978)	Psychoanalysis		New York, 1938
Quadfasel, Alfred (Fred, Fredy) (1902–1981)*	Clinical neurology or neuropsychology		New York, 1936, later Boston
Strauss, Erwin (1891–1975)	Psychiatry		USA, 1938, later Lexington
Jossmann, Paul (1891–1978)	Neuropsychiatry		USA, c. 1938
Schwarz, Hanns (1898–1977)**	Neuropsychiatry		USA (guest lecturer), 1938, return to Berlin, 1939
Kalinowsky, Lothar B. (1899–1992)	"Hallervorden disease"; today pantothenate kinase associated neurodegeneration (prepared for habilitation thesis)		Rome, 1933 London, 1938 New York, 1940
Grotjahn, Martin (1904–1990)*	Psychiatry, psychoanalysis		Topeka, USA, 1937

Note. *Non-Jewish, **Jewish "race report" later revoked.

he was again assisted by Bonhoeffer from 1939–1941, who succeeded in having the Nazi report on his questionable Jewish origin revoked, which saved his and his family's life. In 1946, Schwarz was appointed Director of the Neuropsychiatric Clinic of the University Greifswald in the Soviet Occupied Zone, which later became the German Democratic Republic (GDR; Schwarz, 1975; Gerrens, 2001).

Martin Grotjahn

Dr. Martin Grotjahn (1904–1990) emigrated because of his endangered Jewish wife Etelka Grosz and son Michael to the United States in 1937, first to Topeka, Kansas (Menninger Clinic), and later to Chicago, Illinois. When the war had ended, he and his family moved to Los Angeles, California, in 1945, where he became an influential clinical psychoanalyst.

Herta Seidemann

Herta Seidemann (1900–1984), coworker of Bonhoeffer, conducted extensive studies on "Dyslexia" (Scheller & Seidemann, 1932). However, her habilitation file was not moved forward for her thesis defense by the new National Socialist (NS) authorities at the Berlin Charité. Dr. Seidemann took up an interim position in Switzerland and then returned to Berlin in 1936. On her return, she was presumably hidden by her friends, before she finally immigrated to New York in 1938. This again was aided by Bonhoeffer, who facilitated her emigration by contacting émigré neurologist Kurt Goldstein (1878–1965) at the Montefiore Hospital in Brooklyn, New York. She worked there beginning in 1942 and also joined a psychoanalytical institution, where she collaborated with the German-American émigré psychoanalyst Karen Horney (1885–1952).

Erwin Strauss

Assistant physician and honorary professor Erwin Strauss (1891–1975) continued his tenured job until 1935 because of the "Hindenburg exemption" (Frontkaempfer-Paragraph), by which Jewish men, who had served in the military during WWI, were allowed to stay in their position, but then lost this privilege and the other civil rights through the Nuernberg Race Laws of 1935.

At the beginning of his exile in the United States, he lectured in philosophy and psychology at Black Mountain College in North Carolina. Between 1944 and 1946, he received his license to practice as a physician and became a Research Fellow at Johns Hopkins University, Baltimore, Maryland. He was also Director of the Veterans Administration Hospital in Lexington, Kentucky, from 1946 to 1961 and eventually a lecturer in neurology at the University of Kentucky beginning in 1956. Dr. Strauss resumed his relations with German and Swiss psychiatric colleagues very soon after WWII, in that he lectured in meetings and as guest professor in Frankurt/Main (1952) and Wuerzburg (1961/1962).

Lothar B. Kalinowsky

Lothar B. Kalinowsky (1899–1992) had for some years been a student of the neurologists Richard Cassirer (1868–1925), Paul Schuster (1867–1940), and Karl Bonhoeffer in Berlin.

He prepared his scientific habilitation thesis on "Hallervorden Disease," later substituted by the term "pantothenate kinase-associated neurodegeneration" (Kalinowski, 1936)[2] but then had to leave Berlin and immigrate to Rome in Italy. There, he learned the procedures of electroconvulsive therapy (ECT) from the Italian psychiatrist Ugo Cerletti (1877–1963), with whom he had worked since 1935. After exiles in Paris, France, and Amsterdam, Holland, he immigrated to London, England, in 1938. Kalinowsky left Europe for New York City in 1940. At Columbia University, he became a pioneer of ECT and, in 1958, was promoted to an Associate Professor for Neuropsychiatry at the New York Medical College, while clinically working on the wards of Mount Sinai Hospital.[3]

Paul Jossmann

Paul Jossmann (1891–1978) had been an Adjunct Professor (*Privatdozent*) at Bonhoeffer's clinic since 1929 and one of Bonhoeffer's most experienced and indispensable coworkers. His working contract was prolonged until December 1935 (Gerrens, 2001), when the Nuernberg Race Laws had been enacted. Thereafter, he had to seek refuge in the United States with a letter of recommendation from Bonhoeffer (July 11, 1938), but it took him quite a while to receive a position as an advisory neurologist at the Boston University Medical School and in the Veterans Administration[4] neurology service.

Fred Quadfasel

Fred ("Fredy") Quadfasel (1902–1981) was a resident in Frankfurt/Main during 1925/1926 in the clinic of Kurt Goldstein, who in turn had been a former coworker of Carl Wernicke (1848–1905) but Goldstein's direct contact with Wernicke must have been mostly as a student and for a very short time as his assistant (Quadfasel, 1968). Quadfasel, at the Charitè Hospital Berlin under Bonhoeffer since 1928, had been imprisoned for opposition to the NS regime in November 1934 and was sentenced to two months in jail in February 1935 (Quadfasel, n.d.), before deciding to leave Germany and seeking refuge in the United States. There, he joined the Boston Veterans Administration and was appointed head of the neurological department in 1947 (his impact will be discussed later).

Karl Birnbaum and Franz Josef Kallmann

Two more of Bonhoeffer's former psychiatric collaborators had been expelled from their positions before 1933. Bonhoeffer, through his letters of recommendation to American colleagues facilitated their emigration. However, Prof. Karl Birnbaum (1878–1950) was not allowed to practice due to his lack of a medical license, while Prof. Franz Josef Kallmann (1897–1965) came to lead the Genetics Laboratory of the New York State Psychiatric Institute at Columbia University between 1938 and 1961.

---

[2]The handbook article could yet appear in 1936.
[3]Many of the émigrés, like Dr. Kalinowksi, changed their name either during their forced migration process or at naturalization in their new host countries (e.g., Kalinowsky).
[4]The title of Veterans Administration was the contemporary one for the hospital and medical research system to benefit war-injured soldiers and veterans. It was later renamed and integrated into the Department of Veterans Affairs.

In conclusion, Bonhoeffer's intercessions for his endangered or dismissed coworkers was apparent in at least three directions: (1) to prolong their contracts at the Charité hospital and by declaring them "indispensable" to the clinical work, (2) to help with recommendation letters to foreign colleagues in the host countries, and (3) to use his relations to the higher NS administration and diplomacy for getting passports for Quadfasel or a new "race expert's report" for Schwarz issued. Bonhoeffer's role during the NS period remained nevertheless ambivalent. He took an ambivalent stance towards the eugenics programs of the NS regime and accepted the contemporary sterilization programs, which could be interpreted in line with the *Zeitgeist* among most of the psychiatrists of this time. However, once he was out of office in 1938, Bonhoeffer had to face the even more cruel measures of the Nazi politics. His intercession and aid for his coworkers and émigrés for their settlement in the United States became an instance of noticeable admiration and thankfulness. The former émigrés from his own staff as well as other exiled colleagues in America dedicated an appreciative *Festschrift* for his 80th birthday (March 31, 1948) in an edited collection of 21 papers (Strassmann, 1949: For the great psychiatrist and man who stood firm to his convictions through years of terror and oppression), which appeared shortly after Bonhoeffer's death on December 10, 1948.

Quadfasel's influence on neuropsychology in Boston

The appreciation of Quadfasel's achievements in the Boston's clinical neurology community was expressed by E. Philipp Richardson, Jr. (1924–2013): "Clinical and EEG [Electroencephalography] units at the Veterans Administration Hospitals, esp. that directed by Quadfasel from 1947 to 1964, also played a considerable role" (1975, p. 421). Quadfasel exerted a clear influence on clinical neuropsychology and notable neuropsychologists: Harold Goodglass (1920–2002), later a prominent pioneer of neuropsychological tests and assessment, began his neuropsychological research in the laboratory of Quadfasel. With Quadfasel, he published his first landmark paper (Goodglass & Quadfasel, 1954), in which he showed that the left hemisphere is dominant for language not only in righthanders but also in the majority of lefthanders, thus shaking the classical doctrine that language and handedness are controlled by the same hemisphere (qtd. after Stemmer in Gainotti, 2008, p. XXI; see also, Goodglass, Quadfasel, & Timberlake, 1964).

Quadfasel also influenced Norman Geschwind's (1926–1984) work on aphaseology and neuropsychology and encouraged him to study classical texts of neurology from the nineteenth and early-twentieth century that exposed him to traditional localizationist theory. As Geschwind, who had met Quadfasel in 1958, recalled in his memoirs:

> I would like to express my thanks to two neurologists who grew up under the great German classical tradition, Dr. F. A. Quadfasel, formerly chief of the Neurology Service of the Boston Veterans Administration Hospital, who (together with Dr. Samuel Tartakoff, b. 1903) first provided the author with the opportunity to study a large aphasic population and who constantly provided able criticism and the benefit of profound knowledge of classical writings on aphasia... [And as Geschwind continued: Josephe Jules] Déjerine's [1849–1917] paper, first post-mortem case of pure alexia without agraphia, of which my chief at the Boston VA Hospital Dr. Fred Quadfasel, had an original reprint. The impact of the paper was multiple. (Geschwind, 1974, p. 2)

Geschwind became a founder of modern (behavioral) neuropsychology and the local Aphasia Unit at the Boston Veterans Administration Hospital. He was in line with the classical localizationists ("diagram makers") Carl Wernicke (Kushner, 2015) and referred to earlier papers of German neurologists Hugo Liepmann (1863–1925) and Kurt Goldstein from 1900 to 1909. In particular, Geschwind gathered a sample of observations of so-called disconnection syndromes like pure alexia, color-naming deficits, and motor apraxia, summarized in his work "Disconnection Syndromes in Animals and Man" (Geschwind, 1965a, 1965b), which seemed to have their origin in Quadfasel's library as Geschwind's remembrance implies (Kean, 1994, pp. 351, 356). Quadfasel's own publishing on neurology was not extensive; he figured mostly as a second or third author, such as one with Geschwind on so-called "conduction aphasia" and "isolation of the speech area," supposedly by interruption of the fasciculus arcuatus (Geschwind, Quadfasel, & Segarra, 1968; Kean, 1994).

Exodus from Berlin's independent neurological departments

The disciplinary emancipation of neurology, the beginning of clinical neurology, and the foundation of independent neurological hospital units in Germany happened mainly after WWI, when there was a need to look after the many wounded war veterans. In the prewar years, there existed in Berlin already several outpatient institutions of neurology of a high standard, run mainly by Jewish colleagues like Hermann Oppenheim (1858–1919) who were mostly excluded from academic clinical neurology positions (Holdorff, 2001, pp. 127–139, 2004). Yet during the postwar period, the municipal administration favored the founding of independent hospital units outside of the university. One exception was a special adjunct professorship for neurology and psychiatry at the University of Berlin for Kurt Goldstein, who worked at the academic Hospital of Moabit in Berlin. The neurological avant-garde consisted of a group of Jewish colleagues, who were at the scientific forefront of their time (Holdorff, 2004). Among this particular group figured the following neurological clinical directors:

- Prof. Kurt Goldstein, MD, was born in Kattowitz, Silesia, in 1878 and died in New York City in the United States in 1965 (Neurological Department Berlin-Moabit, 1930–1933).
- Prof. Fritz Heinrich Lewy, MD, was born in Berlin in 1885 and died in Pennsylvania in the United States in 1950 (Neurological Institute, Hansa-Clinic Berlin, 1932–1933).
- Prof. Paul Schuster, MD, was born in Cologne in 1867 and died in London, England, in 1940 (Neurological Department, Friedrich-Wilhelm, or: Hufeland-Hospital Prenzlauer Berg, Berlin, 1920–1933).
- Prof. Clemens Ernst Benda, MD, was born in Berlin in 1898 and died in Munich, Germany, in 1975 (Neurological Department of the Augusta-Hospital Berlin, 1929-1933).
- Otto Maas, MD, was born in Berlin in 1874 and died in London, England, in 1965 (Neurological Department of the Clinic in Berlin-Buch, 1910–1933).
- Kurt Loewenstein, MD, was born in Iserlohn, Germany, in 1894 and died in Tel Aviv, Israel, in 1953 (Neurological Department of the Hospital in Berlin-Lankwitz, 1921–1933).

These Jewish physicians all had to leave their Berlin positions in 1933 and were forced under the Nazi regime to immigrate to other countries outside of Germany, primarily to North America, Britain, and Palestine (Israel). Most of the clinical and research departments, in which they had worked before, disappeared after 1933 or were destroyed during the war (Holdorff, 2004). The assistant medical director (*Oberarzt*) Lipman Halpern (1902–1968), working with Kurt Goldstein at the Moabit Hospital, immigrated first to Switzerland (Zurich).

He later migrated onwards to Palestine, where he was appointed as Head of the Department and Professor of Clinical Neurology at the Hebrew University in Jerusalem (Feinsod, 2012).

Hermann Pineas and Ernst Haase

Hermann Pineas (1892–1969?) served as an assistant medical director in Paul Schuster's clinic and succeeded him from 1939 until 1943 in the director's position of the Jewish Hospital in Berlin. Thereafter, he only survived the Holocaust in Germany through hiding from his Nazi persecutors (Pineas, 1970, 1982). Pineas eventually immigrated to New York when the war had ended, where he took a post as a clinical neurologist from 1952 to 1969 in the Veterans Administration's outpatient clinic. Ernst Haase (1894–1961) had been trained in neurology and psychiatry at several clinics, such as at the Parisian *Salpêtrière* in France with Georges Charles Guillain (1876–1961) and at the Hufeland-Hospital in Berlin with Paul Schuster, before joining Kurt Goldstein at the Moabit Hospital as a medical consultant in 1930. In 1932, however, he returned to youth welfare as well as the care of drug and alcohol addicts (Pross & Winau, 1984). After losing his medical license to practice due to the new Nazi legislation in 1933, he seized on the opportunity to run a private practice as a doctor until October 1939, when he left Germany for England. Eventually, he reached the United States in 1940 where he soon settled in Chicago as a guest physician. In 1941, he passed the State Board Examination and started a private neurological practice. He soon developed contacts to clinical departments in the city, which enabled him to receive an adjunct appointment at the department of neuropsychiatry of the Mount Sinai Hospital from 1941 to 1945. During the same period he also worked in the capacity of a consultant at the Eye and Ear University Clinic in Chicago, Illinois, from 1942. His work then was remunerated with a 20% appointment, which led to an annual salary of $1,500 and allowed for his subsistence. From 1942 to 1947, Haase lectured on neurology at the neuropsychiatric department of the university. After the war, he was appointed as an assistant clinical professor of neurology at the University Clinic of Neurology and Neurosurgery,[5] starting in 1949 in a part-time position with an annual salary of $1,440 (Baule, 1995, p. 129).[6] Haase belonged to the so-called "courtesy staff" at the big municipal Michael Reese Hospital since 1954. With his reaching of retirement age, he was made an adjunct clinician from 1956 to 1958, and, in 1961, shortly before his death, he received the title of an associate attending physician. His scientific papers on neurological and psychotherapeutic topics during the period from 1946 to 1959 display his strong academic engagement (Baule, 1995, p. 129). With the end of the war in 1945, he had held a one-year presidency term of the "executive staff" of the university and, in this position, he became further invited to give talks and addresses to several medical conferences in North America.

Carl Felix List

Carl Felix List (1902–1968) was a German neurologist and neurosurgeon. Following his medical studies in Berlin, he pursued graduate work in neurology in both Berlin and Breslau (of particular importance was his period as a coworker of Paul Schuster in the neurological department of the Hufeland-Hospital in Berlin). In 1932, he

---

[5]Personal files of the "President's Office", University of Illinois, Chicago, qtd. after Baule (1995).
[6]Personal files of the "President's Office", University Illinois in Chicago, cit. after Baule, ibid.

furthermore became a guest surgeon at the Peter Bent Brigham Hospital in New Haven (in neuropathology and neurosurgery with Harvey Cushing) and in Chicago, Illinois, for some months. On his return to Berlin, he trained at Moabit Hospital with the neurosurgeon Moritz Borchardt (1868–1948) until the latter's dismissal in March 1933. Via Brussels, he reached the United States in 1934, where he joined the Department of Neurosurgery in Ann Arbor, Michigan. He also became appointed as a teaching lecturer and received his medical license for neurology and psychiatry before the outbreak of the war. In 1941, he passed the American Board of Psychiatry and Neurology examinations and eventually became a member of the American Neurological Association. When the war had ended, List moved to Grand Rapids, Michigan, in 1946, where he stayed in several clinical positions until his sudden death in 1968, leaving his wife, Eva, a daughter and a son behind. List's clinical focus was on arteriography of the neck vessels and abnormalities of the osseous cervico-occipital region (DeJong, 1970; Davenport, 1993).

The former chiefs of neurological departments from Berlin—Clemens Ernst Benda, Fritz Heinrich Lewy, and Kurt Goldstein—all settled in the United States in very different scientific and clinical fashions.

Clemens Ernst Benda

Clemens Ernst Benda (1898–1975) was a neuropsychiatrist and neuropathologist, who had trained at diverse teaching hospitals in Southern and Northern Germany, as well as in Switzerland. He was a coeditor of the widely read German medical journal *Die Medizinische Welt*, and, from 1929 to 1933, he was the head of neurology at the Augusta-Hospital in Berlin. In 1936, he immigrated to Boston, where he was appointed as the director of the Wallace Research Laboratory for the Study of Mental Deficiency. He also assumed the clinical directorship at Wrentham State School and received educational duties at Harvard Medical School, primarily in the area of psychiatry.[7] Both of his two great studies of 1949 and 1952 (appearing in German in 1960) on mongolism (trisomia 21) and cretinism as well as their influences on developmental psychological disorders, such as oligophrenia and associations with cerebral palsies resulted in Benda's wide acknowledgement in the scientific community, in which he was recognized as one of the founders of child neurology (cf. Ashwal, 1990, pp. 421–426). But his clinical inclination was more towards the field of psychiatry and psychotherapy. Increasingly, Benda became interested in philosophical and Christian-religious topics about which he started to write at length, resulting in several books — primarily monographs written in German between 1932 and 1970.[8] He stayed in close contact with his former countrymen, while dying in 1975 on his last visit in Munich (Yakovlev, 1975).

---

[7] Benda's curriculum vitae: Benda BMSc 96_21Bio in: Francis A. Countway Library of Medicine. Center for the History of Medicine. Harvard Medical Library and Boston Medical Library.

[8] Bibliography see: BendaBMSc96_1Bib in: Francis A. Countway Library of Medicine. Center for the History of Medicine. Harvard Medical Library and Boston Medical Library, and completed until 1970 – by Ulrike Eisenberg, Berlin (unpublished).

Fritz Heinrich Lewy (1885–1950)

The life and work of Fritz Heinrich Lewy in the first decades of the twentieth century has been described in several recent historical articles (Schiller, 2000; Holdorff, 2002, 2006; Rodrigues e Silva et al., 2010; Holdorff, Rodrigues e Silva, & Dodel, 2013) and may be studied there in detail.[9] Lewy's outstanding milestones of his early career were his description of "intracellular eosinophilic inclusion bodies" in Parkinson's disease in Lewandowsky's *Handbook of Neurology* in 1912, the interruption of his neuroscientific work by the obligation of a military officer in WWI, and the founding of the Neurological Research Institute and Clinic at the Hansa Hospital in Berlin in 1932 (Holdorff & Neumaerker, 2002).

Lewy immigrated with his wife to London during the summer of 1933. However, deprived of the opportunity to find a long-term position in Britain, he decided to emigrate again and directed his plans this time to the United States. In Philadelphia, Charles Harrison Frazier (1870–1936), head of the department of neurosurgery at the University of Pennsylvania School of Medicine in Philadelphia eventually offered Lewy a clinical position. Here, in 1934, he started to work as a university consultant neurologist in neurosurgery and a guest professor of neurophysiology. On September 14, 1934, the Lewys made a request for naturalization to the American government. During the process, Lewy changed his name in steps from "Fritz Heinrich Lewy" to "Frederic Henry Lew(e)y." Yet, it took altogether six years, after their initial request, that the Lewys were finally naturalized on June 12, 1940. Before the war, on August 27, 1936, Lewy had received the American medical license to practice. Influenced through their own experiences as refugees from Germany, Lewy and his wife Flora M. Lewy (1892–1961) kept on helping other displaced persons to find positions in the United States (Rodrigues e Silva et al. 2010).

In the search for a successor in 1936 to the neurology professor and head of the Neurological Institute at the University of Pennsylvania, William Gibson Spiller (1863–1940), the committee under its chair, and the American biophysicist Detlev Bronk (1897–1975) had held the prevailing opinion that Germans could not become accustomed to the American way of treating patients, which also excluded Lewy from being considered for this position.[10] Lewy managed to subsist on an annual research award, which was granted to him on June 13, 1935. He received a yearly allocation of $1,000 starting September 17, 1935 for his interesting work in trigeminal research, which eventually led to some papers (Lewy & Grant, 1938; Lewy, Grant, & Groff, 1937, 1940).[11] Assisted by the Emergency Committee in Aid of Displaced Physicians and also by Frazier, Lewy managed to keep an annual salary of $3,000. This was contributed in equal means by the University of Pennsylvania, the Emergency Committee in Aid of Displaced Physicians, as well as the Rockefeller Foundation. It was a relatively comfortable financial arrangement that served to prolong Lewy's unsecured situation in fixed-term contracts for a longer time.

---

[9]Documents from relevant Berlin archives and Lewy's personal files as a displaced scholar in the Archives of the Society for the Protection of Science and Learning at the Bodleian Library in Oxford, England (Holdorff, 2002) have been recently enriched by American sources by Antonio Rodrigues e Silva in his 2014 MD thesis, guided by his mentor, Professor Richard Dodel at the Clinical Department of Neurology of the University of Marburg.

[10]Rockefeller Foundation, talk between Detlev Bronk (1897–1975) and Henry Cuthbert Bazett (1885–1950) on June 8, 1935. Rockefeller Archive 1935, this and the next citations of RF Archives documents from Rodrigues e Silva 2014, pp. 95–98. Rockefeller Foundation Archives, record group 1.1 Projects, series 241A, box 2, folder 19 "University of Pennsylvania – Lewy, F. H. (Refugee, Neurophysiology), 1935-1939" Rockefeller Archive Center, Sleepy Hollow, NY.

[11]Talk with Henry Lewy, August 26, 1935, Rockefeller Archive 1935, record group 1.1 Projects, series 241A, box 2, folder 19.

However, Frazier passed away on July 26, 1936, and Lewy submitted an additional research application to the Rockefeller Foundation (RF) on October 3, 1936, intending to establish a research program to investigate the trigeminal neuralgias and tuberculous meningites. The members of the university committee, Detlev Bronk and the physiologist Henry Cuthbert Bazett (1885–1950), acknowledged Lewy's role in strengthening the neurology service at the university by combining laboratory work and clinical research in the same unit. Nevertheless, the review commission for the RF research application preferred a younger candidate with modern professional training (Bronk 1936). In his assessment of Lewy, Bronk described him as a good clinician yet not a great scientist, suggesting that Lewy should only be offered a part-time position with the university. Bronk would have even rejected Lewy's application if he had been the chair of the committee, but he acknowledged Frazier's previous aid for Lewy "Frazier's death leaves Lewy uncared for" (Bronk, 1936). Lambert from the Rockefeller Foundation's program in psychiatry and psychosomatics concluded in the same sense: "The answer is, I think, that if Frazier had not looked after Lewy no one else would have" (Bronk, 1936, folder 198). The Rockefeller Foundation was eventually informed by Bronk on February 23, 1937, that the Emergency Committee in Aid of Displaced Physicians would support Lewy with an annual sum of $1,500 for the next two years. Additional matching support from the United Jewish Appeal Committee was also assured after a community donation action. This allowed the Rockefeller Foundation to withdraw its support as was also the case for the Emergency Committee in Aid of Displaced Physicians that ended its support for Lewy in 1939 (Rodrigues e Silva, 2014, p. 98).

In the meantime, local Jewish organizations provided Lewy's full annual salary of $3,000, a situation that remained constant until America entered the war. On September 10, 1940, Lewy had complained to the Rockefeller Foundation that, despite his six-year long tenure with the university, he was still in the position of a visiting professor. Yet, this appeal remained unheard by university officials, and Lewy never received a full-time position in the United States. During his university career at the University of Pennsylvania, Lewy also assumed the position of a visiting professor for neuropathology and neuroanatomy until 1949. Between 1943 and 1946, Lewy had been in the US army in the rank of a lieutenant colonel, in the capacity of which he worked as both a physician and medical researcher. The Lawson Hospital in Atlanta, Georgia, was his first station and Lewy afterwards served as the head of the neurology service at the Cushing General Hospital in Framingham, Massachusetts. While at Framingham, he conducted studies on peripheral nerve damage, laying the foundation for the concept of specialty centers largely devoted to the study of injuries of the peripheral nervous system ("Peripheral Nerve Units"). In cooperation with the Pennsylvania neurosurgeon William P. van Wagenen (1897–1961), Lewy built the first "Peripheral Nerve Unit" at the Cushing General Hospital, which was later expanded by the neurologist Barnes Woodhall (1905–1985) from Duke University and the neurosurgeon Roy Glenwood Spurling (1894–1968) at the US Army's Walter Reed Hospital (Denny Brown, Rose, & Sahs, 1975, p. 535). After WWII in 1946, Lewy returned to his position in the department of neurosurgery and neuropathology at the University of Pennsylvania. Hereafter, he travelled to Argentina in 1949 to learn the Hortega method, a specialized histological silver staining technique, which he later successfully applied to the pathological diagnosis of brain tumors. Lewy and his wife converted to the Quaker community as Lewy's mother had already done in 1943, and the family visited regular meetings of the Haverford Quaker community from that point on. In 1949, Lewy retired from university service for health reasons that were caused by diabetes and arteriosclerosis. On October 5, 1950, at the age of 65, Lewey died suddenly due to coronary thrombosis at his summer home in Pennsburg, Pennsylvania; both he and his wife, who died in 1961, are buried in the cemetery of Haverford, Pennsylvania (Holdorff, 2002; Rodrigues e Silva et al., 2010).

During the years of 1908 to 1923, F. H. Lewy was the first researcher to detail the pathological anatomy of Parkinson's disease (PD) leading to his seminal contribution, entitled "Paralysis agitans. Pathol. Anatomie" (1912). In this work, he described the neuronal eosinophilic inclusion bodies in the brainstem, later accomplished by more systematic investigations in 1923. He generally mentioned the widespread pathology but not expressively the inclusion bodies as a hallmark of PD pathology. In spite of the findings of the Russian neuropathologist Konstantin Nikolaevitch Tretiakoff (1892–1958) in 1919, which experimentally determined the significance of the substantia nigra in PD and coining of the term "Corps de Lewy," this research impact had been surprisingly underestimated by Lewy himself (Lewy, 1924). Since his expulsion from Nazi Germany, Lewy had been cut off from his previously successful research on PD. His article from 1942, entitled "Historical Introduction: The Basal Ganglia and their Diseases" seemed to have been intended as a tribute to the bulk of his earlier basic work on PD. Yet, similarly to his first publication, this article largely avoided discussion of the inclusion bodies. However, who ought to have acknowledged his pioneering discovery than Lewy himself? The same holds for his contemporaries, so that the era of the Lewy bodies and Lewy-body-disease came to follow only after Lewy's death in 1950 (Holdorff, 2002; Holdorff, Rodrigues e Silva, & Dodel, 2013).

The various memberships and fellowships that Lewy received in the United States (Rodriguez e Silva, 2014, pp. 10–11) can be seen as representative of Lewy's commitment to clinical neurological research. Among these count his membership in the American Neurological Association, his membership and vice presidency (1938) of the American Association of Neuropathologists, Lewy's membership in the American Physiological Society and the Association for Research in Mental and Nervous Diseases, as well as his chair's position of the neuropathologic section of the American Hospital Association, and the Board of Trustees of the American Academy of Neurology. Likewise, Lewy was a fellow of the American Medical Association, a member of the Philadelphia Physiological Society and the Philadelphia Neurological Society, correspondence member of the Argentinean Society for Normal and Pathological Anatomy, as well as an honorary member of the Argentinean Society for Neurology, Psychiatry, and Neurosurgery, while also holding fellowships in the American College of Physicians and the College of Physicians of Philadelphia.

A letter, dating October 10, 1943 to the secretaries Miss Simpson (see Fig. 1),[12] and another one to Miss Ursell on September 13, 1947 at the Society for the Protection of Science and Learning in London, England, offer some further insights into the scholars'

---

[12]Academic Assistance Council, later Society for Protection of Learning and Science, London, today: Council for Assisting Refugee Academics (CARA), October 10, 1943). Leaf-no 269 FH Lewy file, 'Bodleian Libraries, University of Oxford' (Department of Special Collections, Weston Library, Broad Street, Oxford OX1 3BG.

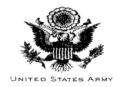

UNITED STATES ARMY

10th October 1943
Lawson General Hosp.
Atlanta. Ga.

Miss Esther Simpson, Secretary.
Soc.f.the Protection of Science.   **19 NOV 1943**
39 Lensfield Road.
Cambridge. England.

Dear Miss Simpson:

          What a nice surprise to receive
to-day your letter and how calming to know that some-
body is trying to straighten out records while we poo
fools are whirling in a maëlstroem of overactivity.

          I am happily settled - as you correctly presume -
in an Army barrack, together with 19 Medical Officers,
certainly in a congenial surrounding since most of us
are professors from various Medical Schools or from
the Rockefeller Institute. I am for quite a while on
leave of absence from my Med.Sch.which is working with
minus almost 100 teachers. I had spent, anyway, most
of the last three years on research in Aviation Medicine for the National Res.Counc.and the Aircorps,aside
from my teaching obligations. At present, the situation is reversed, I am primarily chief of a large neurological service with only eight hours teaching a week
but have still to run investigations for the Aircorps.
Whether I will be able to complete them despite the
continually changing coworkers, is beyond my imagination - possibly after the duration, if there should
be ever such an "after". For the time being, it is my
belief that we few experienced neurologists are much
more needed where the casualties occur and - I am on
the alert. Would'nt it be nice to have lunch together
in the lovely tearoom on the bank of the Cam?

          Mrs.Lewey has returned to Math and computes range
tables for Ordnance in one of the Army's Proving
Grounds, somewhere in the North. My mother keeps
the home fires going and works in the British Relief.

          We hear little of your activities except for
hearing Sir William on his lecture tour. Please, give
my best regards to Adams and. if he should remember
me what I doubt, Professor Gibson. Greetings to you.

                    Sincerely yours.

                    F. H. Lewey.
                    Major M.C., AUS.
                    O -/513965.

Figure 1. Letter to the Academic Assistance Council (Ms. Ursell), dating September 13, 1947. © Reproduced by permission of Bodleian Libraries, University of Oxford (Department of Special Collections, Weston Library, Broad Street, Oxford OX1 3BG).

acculturation overseas and in the US Army. He also mentions in these letter exchanges that he had returned to his former position in the Department of Neuropathology and Neuroanatomy at the University of Pennsylvania in 1946:

> To complete your list: I am now Professor of Neuroanatomy in the Graduate School of Medicine and Associate Professor of Neuropathology in the Medical School of the University of Pennsylvania, and Consultant to the Surgeon General of the Army. A group of our friends over here talked over the scholars we know and who have come to this country since 1933. The general impression is that everybody has found his nook. During the wartime, even older people were gainfully employed.…. Still, I believe that practically everyone makes a living, as small as it may be. The country has been very good to us. (Letter to the Academic Assistance Council (Ms. Ursell), dating September 13, 1947)

In conclusion, in spite of his contentment, Lewy's position at the University of Philadelphia School of Medicine was insecure, and he had to struggle permanently during his American exile. In his first training years in Germany, he had moved between diverse disciplines such as physiology, neuroanatomy, neuropathology, neurology, and internal medicine. Before and after his emigration, his subjects of research ranged widely, a good condition for the directorship of his neurological clinic and research institute in Berlin but perhaps not for finding a firm ground in the host country. He could not profit from his earlier discovery of the inclusion bodies in Parkinson's disease, because he himself and the scientific community were not yet aware of their importance.

Kurt Goldstein (1878–1965) between the natural sciences and humanities

Goldstein was forced to leave Germany in 1933. Having arrived in Berlin from the University of Frankfurt am Main, he had spent only three years at the teaching hospital of Moabit until his arrest and emigration.[13] During his temporary refuge in Amsterdam, he wrote his famous book *Der Aufbau des Organismus. Einfuehrung in die Biologie unter besonderer Beruecksichtigung der Erfahrungen am kranken Menschen* (Goldstein, 1934, 1939) and, hereafter, supported by the Rockefeller Foundation, emigrated to the United States in 1935, where he started to work in private practice. Shortly after his arrival, in 1936, he was appointed as a clinical professor of psychiatry at Columbia University and for some time joined the New York State Psychiatric Institute. He then accepted a position as the chief of the newly founded Laboratory of Neurophysiology at Montefiore Hospital in Brooklyn, where he shifted more to experimental psychology, and, from 1940–1945, he became a clinical professor of neurology at Tufts College Medical School in Boston, Massachusetts. At the age of 67, he then returned to his private practice in New York City and assumed various teaching and educational activities. In the last years of his life, he taught once a week at Brandeis University in Waltham, Massachusetts; however, after suffering from a stroke, he died three weeks later in September 1965.

With his holistic approach to neurology and neuropsychology, Goldstein represented a counterweight to the mainstream of neurological practice. Already during his time in Frankfurt/Main under neuroanatomist Ludwig Edinger (1855–1918) and then being

---

[13]For Goldstein's life and career in Germany, see Hoffmann and Stahnisch (2010), Pow and Stahnisch (2014), and Eling (2012).

Edinger's successor from 1918 to 1930, Goldstein led an institute to study the sequels of traumatic brain injuries — a very innovative program for the rehabilitation of brain-injured patients at this time. Together with Adhémar Gelb (1887–1936), Goldstein also introduced Gestalt psychology into neurology and cofounded the *Internationale Gesellschaft fuer Psychotherapie* [International Society for Psychotherapy] in 1927. Both historical scholars and contemporary neurologists alike have regarded him as an initiator of a multidisciplinary, holistic brain pathology (including aphasiology and neuropsychology), in which psychological, organic, and environmental factors had been inseparable. According to his scientific credo, brain functions could not be individually localized; at best, symptoms and defects could be so diagnosed in neurological diseases and injuries (Goldstein, 1930). A brain-damaged person would lose the ability to proceed from the concrete to the abstract or to distance oneself from the concrete phenomenology of his or her condition and proceed into a world of possibilities to compensate for neurological and behavioral losses received. The concrete attitudes in what Goldstein called the "catastrophic reaction" had thereby to be understood in their dependency as the very individual inner and outer conditions of the individual patients.

Goldstein thereby developed his views about neurological patients from analyses of brain-damaged individuals. He avoided giving additional labeling, primarily of specific brain dysfunctions, since he believed that otherwise the holistic understanding — always considering the whole organism in the practice of neurology—would be lost. He criticized the somatic medicine and psychotherapy. For Goldstein, it was an expression of the atomistic-materialistic way of thinking at the beginning of the twentieth century, which denied the individuality of the personal and social categories (Goldstein, 1931). His debate with Otfrid Foerster (1873–1941) at the Society of German Nerve Doctors (*Gesellschaft Deutscher Nervenaerzte*) on plasticity and regenerative powers in brain-injured patients, which occurred in 1930, offered several insights into the high theoretical and clinical level of the discussion (Holdorff, 1996). It can likewise be seen as an expression of a contemporary crisis in medicine (Rimpau, 2009) due to the schism that appeared between the brain localizationist and holistic approaches. American historian of science Anne Harrington and neurologist Oliver Sacks (1933–2015) have repeatedly stressed Goldstein's view of an "anthropological neurology" in the re-editions of Goldstein's *Der Aufbau des Organismus* (2014) and *The Organism: A Holistic Approach to Biology, Derived from Pathological Data in Man* (1995).[14] The publications from his time in Berlin (1930–1933) reflect a continuation of his earlier work at the University of Frankfurt since WWI. His earlier studies on aphasia were later compiled and republished as a summary volume during his exile in 1948. In view of the skepticism and pragmatism in mainstream American neurology, Goldstein felt the strong need to defend the philosophical implications of his earlier studies on the aphasias (Noppeney, 2000; Noppeney & Wallesch, 2000).

---

[14]"The notion of order is central to Goldstein's ideas of health and disease and those of "rehabilitation: "Thus, being well means to be capable of ordered behavior which may prevail in spite of the impossibility of certain performances which were formerly possible. But the new state of health is not the same as the old one … Recovery is a newly achieved state of ordered functioning … .a new individual norm." Thus, in contradiction to a classical, 'splitting' neurology, Goldstein sees symptoms not as isolated expressions of local damage in the nervous system but as 'attempted solutions' the organism has arrived at, once it has been altered by disease. 'Symptoms,' for Goldstein, betoken whole levels of organization, adaptation to an altered inner state (and world). It is impossible, he emphasizes, to consider any illness – but above all, a neurological illness – without reference to the patient's self, and the forms of his adaptation and orientation within it. Disease, for Goldstein, involves a 'shrinkage' (or, at the least, a 'revision') of self and world, until an equilibrium of a radically new sort can be achieved" (Sacks, 1995, p. 11).

In contrast to his numerous antilocalizationist declarations, his paradoxical linkage to the classical *Hirnpathologie* [brain pathology] and to his teachers Carl Wernicke in Breslau and Edinger in Frankfurt has been noticed by the Boston aphasiologist Norman Geschwind (1926–1984) in an appraisal of Goldstein's role in the history of aphasia research (Geschwind 1965a, 1965b, 1974). To Geschwind, however:

> the most interesting of the four reformers [von Monakow (1853–1930), Pierre Marie (1853–1940), Henry Head (1861–1940), and Goldstein] is Kurt Goldstein, who has actually had much more profound effects on thought about the higher functions, certainly in the United States and probably even in England, than any of the others, even including Head. (Geschwind, 1974, pp. 65–67)

He could never adapt to American culture, and New York remained for him a "home in exile" (Shakow, 1966; and Simmel, 1968, as cited by Noppeney, 2001). In these years, his original writings were almost completely devoted to abstract aspects of psychology and neurology, and he had less impact on current neurology than he deserved (Denny-Brown, 1966). He never managed to take root again or to play as large a role as he had at the height of his earlier career in Germany (Teuber, 1966). The Berlin-born émigré Hans Lukas Teuber (1916–1977), who had met Goldstein in Berlin in familiar conditions as a schoolboy and later became a brilliant neuropsychologist in his own right (Gross, 1994), held tight relations to Goldstein so we owe to him an authentic report of Goldstein (Teuber, 1966). The William James Lectures on Philosophy and Psychology at Harvard during the winter 1938 to 1939, at the invitation from his friend and admirer Karl Spencer Lashley (1890–1958) at Harvard University, were not a success in their oral and written form (Teuber, 1966). With his coinvestigator, the psychologist Martin Scheerer (1900–1961), like him a German émigré, Goldstein developed a test on abstract and concrete behavior to document the individual reactions in brain-injured patients (Goldstein & Scherer, 1941; see also, Henderson, 2010), yet it could not withstand the objections of several neurological and psychological critics. The famous patient Johann Schneider (1891–1962) — traumatized in WWI and studied by Goldstein and his coworker and Gestalt psychologist Adhémar Gelb (Goldstein & Gelb, 1920) — seemed to represent a case of "mind-blindness" ("*Seelenblindheit*").

In later years, however, this patient was reexamined in 1942 in Germany by the neurologists Richard Jung (1911–1986) in 1942 and again by Eberhard Bay (1908–1989) in 1949 with the conclusion that the original disturbances were due to psychological suggestion or swindling on behalf of the patient. Goldstein himself did not accept that he had been "fooled" by his former patient and took the opportunity to visit Schneider again in postwar-Germany and could confirm his original findings (Goldstein 1956). As McDonald Critchley (1900–1992) pointed out, his personal skepticism about Goldstein's famous case darkened their friendly relationship for many years. For him, this showed Goldstein's sensitivity and also inability to distance himself from the conclusions of his paper and the arguments of his critics (Critchley, 1990). Yet up to this day, however, the paradigmatic patient case remains unresolved (Marotta & Behrmann, 2004). In his earlier years in Germany, Goldstein had made many important contributions to mainstream clinical neurology (Benton, 2003). His spectrum of scientific interests included a large number of related disciplines, such as psychotherapy, psychiatry, philosophy, along with neuropsychology and of course neurology, and neuropsychology as well as neurorehabilitation.

In conclusion, Goldstein's expulsion from his home country in 1933 nearly extinguished his influence on German neurological thinking. After his death, several researchers pointed out that he had a lasting impact on American neuropsychology (Teuber, 1966; Eling, 2012) as well as overseas (Luria, 1966), and less on clinical neurology than he deserved (Denny-Brown, 1966). In the view of Iowa psychologist Arthur Lester Benton (1909–2006) four decades later, not all but just a few of his observations and reflections had been accepted by the neurological community. This particularly regards his concept of "abstract attitude" and the "abstract behavior" or symptoms of episodic apathy, stubbornness, and facetiousness as an expression of defensive reactions to protect the patient's self-esteem or to ward off anxiety, following neurological injuries such as stroke (Benton, 2003).

Discussion

The best chances to learn English and to master the professional challenges, following their arrival in North America, had the young undergraduate medical students from Berlin. This is demonstrated by the later Heinz Lehmann[15] (1911–1999) and Fritz A. Freyhan (1912–1982) and the neuropsychologist Hans-Lukas Teuber (1916–1977). The émigré neurologists and psychiatrists, who had formerly worked on Karl Bonhoeffer's staff, were all specialized in the German tradition of neuropsychiatry; their professional settlement often depended on specific local and personal circumstances. Fred Quadfasel and Paul Jossmann were able to continue their work in clinical neurology, while Quadfasel even rose through the ranks to becoming a chief of the neurological department in the Veterans Administration hospital in Boston, Massachusetts. Some could continue their professional work quite smoothly: Psychiatrist Lothar B. Kalinowsky could apply electroconvulsive therapy (ECT) broadly after he had learned this technique with Ugo Cerletti during his previous exile in Rome. Hertha Seidemann found her first refuge in Goldstein's laboratory at the Montefiore Hospital in Brooklyn; Kallmann, following his receipt of a family affidavit, could continue his research program in genetic psychiatry. On the contrary, Erwin Strauss was only able to recommence his clinical psychiatry work after struggling for some years to receive his medical license of practice.

It is beyond the scope of this survey to describe and qualify the émigré physicians in the field of psychiatry in North America as well; yet clearly a noticeable influence could be appreciated. The émigrés from Germany typically combined both neurology and psychiatry in their clinical and research work, as they had been trained in their home country. Not seldom, however, they needed to change their disciplinary orientation, as a reflection of the job offers they were to receive in the United States in both disciplines. German-American psychoanalysts Edith Jacobson (1897–1978) and Martin Grotjahn (1904–1990) from Bonhoeffer's staff, for example, settled again in psychoanalysis. Broader description of the fate of psychoanalysis and psychoanalysts in Germany and their settlement and influence in the United States is presented by Lockot (1985) and respectively by Shorter (1997, pp. 166–189, concerning the Berlin group: p. 167). In accordance with the observations of the Cologne psychiatrist Uwe-Hendrik Peters (1992, 2008), the impact of academically working clinical émigré psychiatrists on British psychiatry was high; in the United States, the émigré psychoanalysts dominated psychiatry, increasingly after WWII (Shorter 1997, pp. 166–169).

---

[15]The working situation of Heinz Lehmann is further described in the article by Stahnisch (2016) in this special issue.

The former avant-garde of clinical neurology in Berlin consisted of highly qualified neurologists, who frequently could not resume their former clinical and research directions field or only to a minor degree: for example, Kurt Goldstein or Frederic Henry Lewy (Denny-Brown, 1966; Teuber, 1966; Rodrigues e Silva et al. 2010; Holdorff, Rodrigues e Silva, and Dodel 2013). The struggle for their resettlement in North America was enormous and sometimes even deploring. Lewy could himself rely on the aid and tutelage of the acquainted neurosurgeon Charles Harrison Frazier (1870–1936) in Philadelphia, help from the Rockefeller Foundation, the Emergency Committee in Aid of Displaced Scholars, and eventually also on local Jewish community funds. However, at the university, he never reached his former level of clinical neurology work and research again. This appears to have had several reasons: Before his forced migration from Berlin, he had struggled to found and head a neurological clinic and research institute until its final opening in 1932. His neuroscientific activities were multiple and spanned neuropathology, neuroanatomy, and clinical neurology, yet they were too broad for a new start overseas. His plan to begin an altered research program on the trigeminal neuralgias was not a promising one. His claim to fame, as the discoverer of the "inclusion bodies" in Parkinson's disease (Lewy, 1912), was itself a development that rather ensued after his death — even Lewy himself had not fully recognized its importance. The fact that German-Jewish neurologists and neuroscientists used to pursue their rotations and postgraduate training in Germany in several clinics and laboratories before the war appears to have hampered their professional resettlement in America. Goldstein pursued widely diversified topics with little interrelation. He seemingly scattered his efforts, often as a reflection of the sheer necessities of daily practical problems in the medical field of his new host country (Goldstein, 1967). His impact on mainstream neurology was much less than that on neuropsychology and anthropology. Neuropsychology generally plays a larger role in the diagnostic process of special cases and employs laboratory studies and theoretical considerations than did contemporary neurology. Neuropsychiatrist Clemens Ernst Benda had a much better start in Boston as a clinical fellow. Very soon he became appointed as the head of an institution for "feeble-minded" and handicapped children, where he gathered extensive clinical and neuropathological data that led to two important books on trisomia 21 and cretinism as well as developmental disorders. This later credited him a place as one of the founders of child neurology in North America. Other émigré neurologists from Berlin resettled successfully in medium-sized American hospitals and clinics: Carl Felix List, Ernst Haase, and Hermann Pineas can be seen as respective examples of this group.

A very different integration process into the professional and cultural life of American society can be seen in the cases of two non-Berlin scholars: the neurologists Alfred Hauptmann from the University in Halle/Saale and Robert Wartenberg from Freiburg University. The overseas conditions for their emigration to the U.S. were much better for Wartenberg due to his knowledge of the language and the acquaintance with American clinics from his previous Rockefeller fellowship in 1925/1926. Also a new house in San Francisco was immediately available for the Wartenberg family at their arrival (Rosenow, Dietz, and Frowein, 2007). Robert Wartenberg was a Russian-born, German-educated professor of neurology from the German University Freiburg, where he had served at the Department of Neurology for almost 15 years.[16] At the end of 1935, he immigrated to New York, and, in April

[16]His teachers in neurology were Alfred Hoche (1865–1943), Otfrid Foerster (1873–1941), Richard Cassirer (1868–1925), and Max Nonne (1861–1959). For further biographical details and references (obituaries), see Rosenow, Dietz, and Frowein (2007).

1935, he and his family moved to San Francisco where his wife's relatives owned private property. Under the tutelage of the neurologist Bernard Sachs (1858–1946) and with the aid of the biochemist Daniel E. Koshland (1920–2007) along with the local neurosurgeon Howard Naffziger (1884–1961), he received an academic position at the University of California School of Medicine at San Francisco. Here, however, he faced several conflicts with the Neuropsychiatric Division of the Department of Medicine, since Wartenberg's interests collided with those of the other division in which psychiatry and neurology were likewise integrated under one roof as well, which was fairly unusual in the US medical schools of the time (Aird, 1988). As American child neurologist Roger Baker Aird recalled:

> Except for the generous and continuing local support of refugee funds, plus the intervention of us, Wartenberg could not have survived for long in this precarious situation. (Aird, 1994, p. 24)

Aird's personal reminiscences on Wartenberg, as well as on other German émigrés' teaching of neurology reflect insightful observations as well as problematic generalizations at the same time in that he concluded from Wartenberg's "bombastic" "showman's" teaching to the German medical teaching with its "primadonnas," who ignore "the more realistic experience of patient workups and follow through with their complex problems" (Aird, 1994, pp. 223–224). However, Wartenberg's personality and teaching skills have been lauded by other observers (Denny Brown, Rose, & Sahs, 1975, p. 491; Schiller, 2003, p. 80). Aird's successor Robert Fishman (1924–2012) stated in a personal communication: "Wartenberg was the first well-trained neurologist in Northern California," but, concerning Wartenberg's influence in US-American neurology, "There were so many other neurologists of his generation who had a greater impact" (Fishman to Rosenow 2005, cit. in Rosenow, Dietz, & Frowein, 2007, p. 449). His textbooks on "Reflexes" and "Diagnostic Tests in Neurology" became very popular in American and German Neurology (Wartenberg, 1945, 1953, 1958a; see also, Boes, 2015; Maranhão-Filho, Borges Vincent, & Martins da Silva, 2015; Wartenberg, 1958b). In honoring his work, several eponyms still bear his name, such as "Wartenberg's Disease" and "Wartenberg's Sign,"[17] and the regular Robert Wartenberg Lectures are given at the annual meetings of the American Academy of Neurology, while the bestowment of the Robert Wartenberg Prize in Germany is a tribute to his enduring memory in his former homeland.

In contrast to these instances of a successful integration of the above-mentioned neurologists in North America stands the tragic fate of Alfred Hauptmann (1881–1948). He was more a clinical neurologist than a psychiatrist and was well accepted for his studies on phenobarbital therapy in epilepsy. Hauptmann was expulsed from his chair of psychiatry at the University of Halle and was imprisoned in the concentration camp Dachau for several weeks in 1935 before he could eventually flee to Switzerland. Lacking a medical license to practice, he emigrated on to London, England, and finally to Boston, Massachusetts, in the United States in October 1939. There he joined the Joseph Pratt Diagnostic Hospital as an advisory neurologist, and together with a fellow émigré physician, the internist Siegfried Joseph Thannhauser (1885–1962) he described a dominant hereditary myopathy, later credited with the eponym Hauptmann-Thannhauser myopathy

---

[17]Wartenberg's disease (syn.: Cheiralgia paresthetica): A sensitive neuropathy involving the superficial branch of the radial nerve; Wartenberg's sign: In ulnar paralysis the little finger is in a position of abduction; Wartenberg's syndrome: Radial nerve entrapment at the forearm; Wartenberg wheel: A medical device for neurological use. Wartenberg's migratory sensory neuropathy: A benign, relapsing and remitting condition.

(Hauptmann & Thannhauser, 1941). However, Hauptmann was already 58 years of age and could never accept his exile. On April 5, 1948, he seemed to have died of a "broken heart" (Obituary of his widow Selma Hauptmann, as qtd. in Kumbier & Haack, 2002).

The neurological scholars, expelled from their clinical work in Berlin, were mostly integrated into the new scientific communities of their host countries, as the examples of Clemens Ernst Benda, Kurt Goldstein, Frederic Henry Lewy, and Robert Wartenberg show. They, including psychiatrist Lothar Bruno Kalinowsky, contributed to the great sample of Webb Haymaker's and Francis Joseph Schiller's "Founders of Neurology" (1953 (2nd ed.), 1970). The editors Haymaker, a previous visiting scientist in Europe, and Schiller, also an émigré physician from Europe himself, both held the European founders of neurology in high esteem. In the official historical survey of the centennial anniversary of American neurology in the 1970s (Merritt and other contributors in Denny Brown, Rose, & Sahs, 1975), however, Lewy was only mentioned for his foundation of a peripheral nerve unit during WWII, Wartenberg for his clinical and educational contributions, and Quadfasel for his considerable role at the Boston Veterans Administration Hospital (Richardson, 1975). None of them were included in the "History of 20th Century Neurology" (Tyler et al., 2003a, 2003b), which shows that their biographies and important contributions to American neurology had largely fallen into obscurity in the American neurological community. Nevertheless, as this article has shown, their contributions and achievements can still be identified and appraised in the neurological eponym of the Lewy bodies, the Wartenberg signs, Benda's impact as one of the founders of child neurology, as well as in the continuous discussions regarding Goldstein's contributions to neuropsychology, rehabilitation neurology, anthropology, and philosophy.

References

Aird RB (1988): Some reminiscences. *Archives of Neurology* 45: 1145–1155.

Aird RB (1994): *Foundations of Modern Neurology: A Century of Progress.* New York, Raven Press.

Ashwal S (1990): *The Founders of Child Neurology.* San Francisco, Norman Publisher.

Baule C (1995): *Ernst Haase (1894–1961): Neurologe, Psychiater, Psychotherapet, Sozialmediziner. Sein Leben und Werk.* PhD Dissertation. Berlin, Free University.

Bay E, Lauenstein O, Cibis P (1949): Ein Beitrag zur Frage der Seelenblindheit. Der Fall Schn. Von Gelb und Goldstein. *Psychiatrie, Neurologie, und Medizinische Psychologie* 1: 73–91.

Benda CE (1949): *Mongolism and Cretinism.* New York, Heinemann, 2nd revised edition.

Benda CE (1952): *Developmental Disorders of Mentation and Cerebral Palsies.* New York, Heinemann.

Benton A (2003): Recollections of a part-time amateur historian. *Journal of the History of the Neurosciences* 12: 25–33.

Boes CJ (2015): History of neurologic examination books. *Proceedings of the Baylor University Medical Center* 28: 172–179.

Bronk D (1936, October 29): Rockefeller Archive 1936, record group 1.1 Projects, series 241A, box 2, folder 19.

Critchley M, ed. (1990): Kurt Goldstein. In: *The Ventricle of Memory.* New York, Raven Press, pp. 72–83.

Davenport HW (1993): *University of Michigan Surgeons, 1850–1970: Who They Were and what They Did.* Ohio, MI, University of Michigan Libraries.

DeJong RN (1970): Carl Felix List 1902–1968. *Transactions of the American Neurological Association* 95: 339.

Denny-Brown D (1966): The organismic (holistic) approach: The neurological impact of Kurt Goldstein. *Neuropsychologia* 4: 293–297.

Denny Brown AS, Rose ALS, Sahs AL, eds. (1975): *Centennial Anniversary Volume of the American Neurological Association 1875–1975*. New York, Springer.

Duggan ST (1941/1987): Annual report of the Emergency Committee in Aid of Displaced Foreign Scholars. In: Strauss HA, Buddensieg T, Duewell HK, eds., *Emigration. Deutsche Wissenschaftler nach 1933. Entlassung und Vertreibung*. Berlin, Technische Universitaet Berlin, Teil III, pp. 1–4.

Eling P (2012): Neurognostic answer: Kurt Goldstein. *Journal of the History of the Neurosciences* 21: 121–125.

Feinsod M (2012): The neurologist Lipman Halpern—Author of the Oath of the Hebrew Physician. *Rambam Maimonides Medical Journal* 3 (epublication ahead of print).

Fijal A (1994): Die Rechtsgrundlagen der Entpflichtung juedischer und politisch missliebiger Hochschullehrer nach 1933 sowie des Umbaus im nationalsozialistischen Sinne. In: Fischer W, Hierholzer K, Hubenstorf M, Walther P, Winau R, eds., *Exodus der Wissenschaften aus Berlin*. Berlin, De Gruyter, pp. 101–115.

Gainotti G (2008): Prologue. In: Stemmer B, Whitaker HA, eds., *Handbook of the. Neuroscience of Language*. Oxford, Academic Press Elsevier, p. xxi.

Gerrens U (2001): Psychiater unter der NS-Diktatur. Karl Bonhoeffers Einsatz fuer rassisch und politisch verfolgte Kolleginnen und Kollegen. *Fortschritte der Neurologie und Psychiatrie* 69: 330–339.

Geschwind N (1964): The paradoxical position of Kurt Goldstein in the history of aphasia. *Cortex* 1: 214–224.

Geschwind N (1965a): Disconnexion syndromes in animals and man. I. *Brain* 88: 237–294.

Geschwind N (1965b): Disconnexion syndromes in animals and man. II. *Brain* 88: 585–644.

Geschwind N (1974): *Selected Papers on Language and the Brain*. Dordrecht, Holland, Boston, D. Riedel Publishing Company.

Geschwind N, Quadfasel FA, Segarra JM (1968): Isolation of the speech area. *Neuropsychologia* 6: 327–340.

Goldstein K (1930): Die Restitution bei Schaedigungen der Hirnrinde. *Deutsche Zeitschrift fuer Nervenheilkunde* 116: 2–26.

Goldstein K (1931): Das psychophysische Problem in seiner Bedeutung fuer aerztliches Handeln. *Therapie der Gegenwart* 72: 1–11.

Goldstein K (1934): *Der Aufbau des Organismus. Einfuehrung in die Biologie unter besonderer Beruecksichtigung der Erfahrungen am kranken Menschen*. Den Haag, Nijhoff.

Goldstein K (1939): *The Organism: A Holistic Approach to Biology, Derived from Pathological Data in Man*. New York, American Book Company.

Goldstein K (1956): Bemerkungen zur Methodik der Untersuchung psychopathologischer Faelle – Im Anschluss an die Nachuntersuchung des seelenblinden Patienten Schneider, mehr als 30 Jahre nach dem Auftreten der Stoerung. *Monatsschrift fuer Psychiatrie und Neurologie* 131: 309–336.

Goldstein K (1967): Kurt Goldstein (ed. by Riese W). In: Boring E, Lindzey G, eds., *A History of Psychology in Autobiography*. New York, Appleton-Century-Crofts, pp. 148–166.

Goldstein K (1995): *The Organism: A Holistic Approach to Biology, Derived from Pathological Data in Man*. New York, Zone Books, English edition.

Goldstein K (2014): *T Der Aufbau des Organismus*, Hoffmann T, Stahnisch FW, Begleitwort Anne Harrington, eds. Paderborn, Wilhelm Finke Verlag, German edition.

Goldstein K, Gelb A, eds. (1920): *Psychologische Analysen hirnpathologischer Faelle*. Leipzig, J. Barth.

Goldstein K, Scherer M (1941): *Abstract and Concrete Behavior: An Experimental Study with Special Tests*. Evanston, IL, American Psychological Association.

Goodglass H, Quadfasel FA (1954): Language laterality in left-handed aphasics. *Brain* 77: 521–548.

Goodglass H, Quadfasel FA, Timberlake WH (1964): Phrase length and the type and severity of aphasia. *Cortex* 7: 133–155.

Gross C (1994): Hans-Lukas Teuber: A tribute. *Cerebral Cortex* 5: 451–454.

Hauptmann A, Thannhauser SJ (1941): Muscular shortening and dystrophy: A heredofamilial disease. *Archives of Neurology and Psychiatry* 46: 654–664.

Haymaker W, Schiller F (1970): *The Founders of Neurology*. Springfield, IL, Charles C Thomas, 2nd edition.

Hécaen H (1979): H.-L. Teuber et la fondation de la neurologie expérimentale. *Neuropsychologia* 17: 199–224.

Henderson VW (2010): Cognitive assessment in neurology, in particular on executive functions with special tests of abstract behavior, developed by Goldstein and Scheerer and his colleagues (tab. 17.3, p. 24), and stick-test (fig. 17.8, p. 249). In: Finger S, Boller F, Tyler KL, eds., *History of Neurology: Handbook of Neurology*. Edinburgh, Elesiver, Vol. 95, pp. 235–256.

Holdorff B (1996): Die Lokalisationsdiskussion vor 60 Jahren (O. Foerster, K. Goldstein, V. v. Weizsaecker). *Schriftenreihe der Deutschen Gesellschaft fuer Geschichte der Nerven-heilkunde* 1: 139–142.

Holdorff B (2001): Die nervenärztlichen Polikliniken in Berlin vor und nach 1900. In: Holdorff B, Winau R, eds., *Geschichte der Neurologie in Berlin*. Berlin, De Gruyter, pp. 127–139.

Holdorff B (2002): Friedrich Heinrich Lewy (1885–1950) and his work. *Journal of the History of the Neurosciences* 11: 19–28.

Holdorff B (2004): Founding years of clinical neurology in Berlin until 1933. *Journal of the History of the Neurosciences* 13: 223–238.

Holdorff B (2006): Fritz Heinrich Lewy (1885–1950). *Journal of Neurology* 253: 677–678.

Holdorff B, Neumaerker KJ (2002): Die Geschichte des von F. H. Lewy 1932 gegruendeten neurologischen Instituts in Berlin. *Schriftenreihe der Deutschen Gesellschaft fuer Geschichte der Nervenheilkunde* 8: 77–96.

Holdorff B, Rodrigues e Silva AM, Dodel R (2013): Centenary of Lewy bodies (1912–2012). *Journal of Neural Transmission* 120: 509–516.

Hurvich LM, Jameson D, Rosenblith WA (1987): Hans-Lukas Teuber: A biographical memoir. *Biographical Memoirs, National Academy of Sciences* 57: 461–490.

Jung, R (1949): Ueber eine Nachuntersuchung des Falles Schn … von Goldstein und Gelb. *Psychiatrie, Neurologie und Medizinische Psychologie* 1: 352–362.

Kalinowski L (1936): Hallervordensche Krankheit. In: Bumke O, Foerster O, eds. *Handbuch der Neurologie*, Band 16. Berlin, Springer Berlin, pp. 874–881.

Kater MH (1989): *Doctors under Hitler*. Chapel Hill, The University of North Carolina Press.

Kean, M-L (1994): Introduction to Norman Geschwind. In: Eling P, ed., *Reader in the History of aphasia: From [Franz] Gall to [Norman] Geschwind*. Amsterdam, John Benjamins, p. 351, 356.

Kramer F, Pollnow H (1930): Symptomenbild und Verlauf einer hyperkinetischen Erkrankung im Kindesalter. *Allgemeine Zeitschrift fuer Psychiatrie* 96: 214–216.

Kramer F, Pollnow H (1932): Ueber eine hyperkinetische Erkrankung im Kindesalter. *Monatsschrift fuer Psychiatrie und Neurologie* 82: 2–39.

Kroener HP (1988): Die Emigration von Medizinern unter dem Nationalsozialismus. *Deutsches Aerzteblatt* 85: 2573–2578.

Kumbier E, Haack K (2002): Alfred Hauptmann – Schicksal eines deutsch-juedischen Neurologen. *Fortschritte der Neurologie und Psychiatrie* 70: 204–209.

Kushner HI (2015): Norman Gewchwind and the use of history in the (re)birth of behavioral neurology. *Journal of the History of the Neurosciences* 24: 173–192.

Lewy FH (1912): Paralysis agitans. Pathol. Anatomie. In: Lewandowsky K, ed., *Handbuch der Neurologie*. Bd. III, spez. Neurol. II. Berlin, Springer, pp. 920–933.

Lewy FH (1923): *Die Lehre vom Tonus und der Bewegung. Zugleich systematische Untersuchungen zur Klinik, Physiologie, Pathologie und Pathogenese der Paralysis agitans*. Berlin, Springer.

Lewy FH (1924): Paralysis agitans. In: Kraus F, Brugsch T, eds., *Spezielle Pathologie und Therapie innerer Krankheiten*. Berlin, Urban Schwarzenberg Verlag, pp. 697–750.

Lewy FH (1942): Historical introduction: The basal ganglia and their diseases. In: Putnam TJ, Frantz AM, Ranson SE, eds., *The Diseases of the Basal Ganglia*. Baltimore, Williams and Wilkens, pp. 1–20.

Lewy FH, Grant FC, Groff RA (1937): Representation of autonomic innervation of head in mesencephalic trigeminus nucleus. *Transactions of American Neurological Association* 63: 140–143.

Lockot R, ed. (1985): *Erinnern und Durcharbeiten. Zur Geschichte der Psychoanalyse und Psychotherapie im Nationalsozialismus*. Frankfurt a. M., Fischer.

Luria AR (1966): Kurt Goldstein and neuropsychology. *Neuropschologia* 4: 311–313.

Maranhão-Filho P, Borges Vincent M, Martins da Silva M (2015): Exame neurológico: autores pioneiros e seus livros. *Arqiva Neuro-Psiquiatrica* (São Paulo) 73. Retrieved from http://www.scielo.br/scielo.php?pid=S0004-282X2015000200140&script=sci_arttext

Marotta JJ, Behrmann M (2004): Patient Schn.: Has Goldstein and Gelb's case withstood the test of time? *Neuropsychologia* 42: 633–638.

Milner B, Teuber HL (1968): Alteration of perception and memory in man: Reflections on methods. In: Weiskrantz L, ed., *Analysis of Behavioral Change*. New York: Harper & Row, pp. 274–328.

Neumaerker KJ (2005): The Kramer-Pollnow-syndrome: A contribution on the life and work of Franz Kramer and Hans Pollnow. *History of Psychiatry* 16: 435–451.

Noppeney U (2000): *Abstrakte Haltung: Kurt Goldstein im Spannungsfeld von Neurologie, Psychologie und Philosophie*. Wuerzburg, Koenigshausen und Neumann, pp. 23–24.

Noppeney U (2001): Kurt Goldstein – A philosophical scientist. *Journal of the History of the Neurosciences* 10: 67–78.

Noppeney U, Wallesch C (2000): Language and cognition—Kurt Goldstein's theory of semantics. *Brain and Cognition* 44: 367–386.

Pearle KM (1981): *Preventive Medicine: The Refugee Physician and the New York Medical Community 1933–1945*. Working papers on blocked alternatives in the health policy system. Bremen, University of Bremen.

Peiffer J (1998): Die Vertreibung deutscher Neuropathologen. *Nervenarzt* 69: 99–109.

Peters UH (1992): *Psychiatrie im Exil*. Kupka, Verlag Duesseldorf.

Peters UH (2008): Emigrierte Berliner Psychiatrie. In: Helmchen H, ed., *Psychiater und Zeitgeist: Zur Geschichte der Psychiatrie in Berlin*. Lengerich, Pabst, pp. 305–317.

Pineas H (1970): Meine aktive Verbundenheit mit dem juedischen Sektor Berlins. In: Strauss HA, Grossmann KR, eds., *Gegenwart im Rueckblick*. Heidelberg, Stiehm, pp. 299–301.

Pineas H (1982): Unsere Schicksale seit dem 30. Januar 1930. In: Richardz M, ed., *Juedisches Leben in Deutschland. Selbstzeugnisse zur Sozialgeschichte 1918–1945*. Stuttgart, Deutsche Verlagsanstalt, pp. 429–442.

Poeck K (1982): *Klinische Neuropsychologie*. Stuttgart, Thieme.

Pow S, Stahnisch FW (2014): Kurt Goldstein (1878–1965) – Pioneer in Neurology. *Journal of Neurology* 261: 1049–1050.

Pross C, Winau R, eds. (1984): *"Nicht misshandeln". Das Krankenhaus Moabit*. Berlin, Edition Hentrich, pp. 122–130.

Quadfasel F (n.d.): Personal file of Fredy Quadfasel, Humboldt-Universitaetsarchiv, Akte Charité-Krankenhaus, Charité PA 26, Bd.133, PA Med.1, Quadfasel Fredy, pp. 28–29.

Quadfasel F (1968): Aspects of the life and work of Kurt Goldstein. *Cortex* 4: 113–124.

Richardson EP, Jr. (1975): A history of neurology in Boston. In: Denny Brown AS, Rose ALS, eds., *Centennial Anniversary Volume of the American Neurological Association 1875–1975*. New York, Springer, pp. 413–421.

Rimpau W (2009): Die Krise der Neurologie in erkenntnistheoretischer Weise: Kontroverse zwischen Viktor von Weizsaecker, Kurt Goldstein und Otfrid Foerster zum Lokalisationsprinzip. *Nervenarzt* 80: 970–974.

Rodrigues e Silva AM (2014): *Biographie und wissenschaftliche Arbeiten von Prof. Dr. Fritz Heinrich Lewy (1885–1950)*. MD thesis. Marburg, Philipps-University.

Rodrigues e Silva AM, Geldsetzer F, Holdorff B, Kielhorn FW, Balzer-Geldsetzer M, Oertel WH, Hurtig H, Dodel R (2010): Who was the man who discovered the "Lewy bodies"? *Movement Disorders* 25: 1765–1773.

Rosenow DE, Dietz H, Frowein R (2007): Robert Wartenberg (19.06.1886–16.11.1956). Ein Entwurzelter der Deutschen Neurologie. *Schriftenreihe der Deutschen Gesellschaft fuer Nervenheilkunde* 13: 429–459.

Rothenberger A, Neumaerker KJ (2005): *Wissenschaftsgeschichte der ADHS – Kramer-Pollnow im Spiegel der Zeit*. Steinkopf, Darmstadt.

Sacks O (1995): Foreword. In: Goldstein K, ed., *The Organism: A Holistic Approach to Biology, Derived from Pathological Data in Man*. New York, Zone Books, pp. 7–14.

Scheller H, Seidemann H (1932): Zur Frage der optisch-räumlichen Agnosie. pp. 97–116. Zugleich ein Beitrag zur Dyslexie. *Mschr Psychiat Neurol* 81: 97–116.

Schiller F (2000): Fritz Lewy and his bodies. *Journal of the History of the Neurosciences* 9: 148–151.

Schiller F (2003): An autobiographical sketch. *Journal of the History of the Neurosciences* 12: 76–84.

Schwarz H (1975): *Jedes Leben ist ein Roman*. Berlin, Buchverlag der Morgen.

Shorter E (1997): *A History of Psychiatry: From the Era of Asylums to Prozac*. London, John Wiley & Sons, Inc.

Stahnisch FW (2008): Zur Zwangsemigration deutschsprachiger Neurowissenschaftler nach Nordamerika: Der historische Fall des Montreal Neurological Institute. *Schriftenreihe der Deutschen Gesellschaft fuer Geschichte der Nervenheilkunde* 14: 441–472.

Stahnisch FW (2016): Learning soft skills the hard way: Historiographical considerations on the cultural adjustment process of German-speaking émigré neuroscientists in Canada, 1933 to 1963. *Journal of the History of the Neurosciences* 25: 299–319.

Strassmann G (1949): For the great psychiatrist and man who stood firm to his convictions through years of terror and oppression. *Monatsschrift fuer Psychiatrie und Neurologie* 117: 360–366.

Strauss HA, Buddensieg T, Duewell K, eds. (1987): *Emigration. Deutsche Wissenschaftler nach 1933. Entlassung und Vertreibung*. Berlin, Technische Universitaet Berlin.

Teuber HL (1965): Postscript: Some needed revisions of the classical views of agnosia. *Neuropsychologia* 3: 371–378.

Teuber HL (1966): Kurt Goldstein's role in the development of Neuropsychology. *Neuropsychologia* 4: 299–310.

Teuber HL (1978). The brain and human behavior. In: Held R, Leibowitz HW, Teuber HL, eds., *Handbook of Sensory Physiology*. New York, Springer, Volume 7, pp. 879–920.

Teuber HL, Battersby WS, Bender M (1960): *Visual Field Defects After Penetrating Missile Wounds of the Brain*. Cambridge, MA: Harvard University Press.

Tyler K, York GK, Steinberg DA (2003a): History of 20th century neurology: Decade by decade. *Deutsche Zeitschrift fuer Nervenheilkunde* 115: 2–314.

Tyler K, York GK, Steinberg DA (2003b): History of 20th century neurology: Decade by decade. *Deutsche Zeitschrift fuer Nervenheilkunde* 116: 28–31 and 42–45.

Wartenberg R (1945): *The Examination of Reflexes: A Simplification*. Chicago, The Year Book Publishers.

Wartenberg R (1953): *Diagnostic Tests in Neurology*, trans. by H Koebcke. Chicago, The Year Book Publishers.

Wartenberg R (1958a): *Neurologische Untersuchungsmethoden in der Sprechstunde*. Stuttgart, Thieme Verlag.

Wartenberg R (1958b): *Neuritis, Sensory Neuritis, Neuralgia*. New York, Oxford University Press.

Yakovlev PI (1975): Clemens Ernst Benda 1898–1975. *Journal of Neuropathology & Experimental Neurology* 34: 549–550.

Zeidman LA, Kondziella D (2012): Neuroscience in Nazi Europe (Part III): Victims of the Third Reich. *Canadian Journal for the Neurological Sciences* 39: 729–746.

Learning soft skills the hard way: Historiographical considerations on the cultural adjustment process of German-speaking émigré neuroscientists in Canada, 1933 to 1963

Frank W. Stahnisch

ABSTRACT

This article is a historiographical exploration of the special forms of knowledge generation and knowledge transmission that occur along local cultural boundaries in the modern neurosciences. Following the inauguration of the so-called "Law on the Re-Establishment of a Professional Civil Service" in Nazi Germany on April 7, 1933, hundreds of Jewish and oppositional neurologists, neuropathologists, and psychiatrists were forced out of their academic positions, having to leave their home countries and local knowledge economies and traditions for Canada and the United States. A closer analysis of their living and working conditions will create an understanding of some of the elements and factors that determined the international forced migration waves of physicians and clinical neuroscientists in the twentieth century from a historiographical perspective. While I am particularly looking here at new case examples regarding the forced migration during the National Socialist period in Germany, the analysis follows German-speaking émigré neurologists and psychiatrists who found refuge and settled in Canada. These individuals form an understudied group of refugee medical professionals, despite the fact that the subsegments of refugee neurologists and clinical psychoanalysts in the United States, for example, have been a fairly well-investigated population, as the works of Grob (1983), Lunbeck (1995), or Ash and Soellner (1996) have shown. This article is primarily an exploration of the adjustment and acculturation processes of several highly versatile and well-rounded German-speaking physicians, who had received their prior education in neurology, psychiatry, and basic brain research. They were forced out of their academic home institutions and had to leave their clinical research fields as well as their disciplinary self-understanding behind on the other side of the Atlantic.

Introduction

In the recent past, even many historians of medicine and science have endorsed the widespread belief that the exodus of Central European scientists and physicians during the Nazi Period could readily be described in terms of a linear equation of the subtractions and additions of intellect. This common interpretation has simplistically viewed the massive exodus of academics, intellectuals, and scientists after 1933 as an "enrichment" primarily of the North American and British medical and academic communities (see Medawar & Pyke, 2001 or Cornwell, 2003, for example). Although such a perspective is not entirely wrong when a rather quantitative "meta-perspective" is taken, it becomes less compelling when the individual biographies of the respective physicians and scientists themselves are taken into account and are placed in their contingent work environments. This includes their work situations, skill sets, along with the personal and psychological resources of each émigré neuroscientist (cf. Stahnisch, 2010).

This contribution introduces some of those local and cultural factors which implicated the arrival, acceptance, and integration of many German-speaking émigrés doctors and brain researchers into Canada, following their exile between 1933 and 1945, which have largely gone unnoticed by the relevant scholarship on twentieth-century history of neuroscience. When tracing their career paths into the 1960s, during which the scientific research landscapes in Canadian biomedicine gradually came to change with the creation of the Medical Research Council (MRC), the complex cultural modes and scientific interchanges associated with the forced migration process become fairly obvious (MRC, 2000). As the main title ("Learning Soft Skills the Hard Way") of this article implies, the integration of German-speaking émigrés neuroscientists cannot simply be perceived in terms of a supplementation of longstanding North American scientific traditions but needs to be viewed as a very complex process of acculturation on multiple levels of the social and cultural organization of contemporary Canadian and American research landscapes. It is further more of a seemingly modern interest in the cultural makeup of science to analyze and understand the process of forced migration in the neuroscientific field while mapping the often drastic changes that took place to the career patterns of this particular group of medical professionals (Zeidman, 2014). Based on the existing historical evidence, the traditional views on the forced migration process in the neurosciences and psychiatry need to be significantly readjusted and refined.

Situating a cultural view in the historiography of forced migration in the neurosciences

Although most core facts about the exodus of medical researchers during the period of Nazism in Germany are already known (cf. Seidelman, 2000, pp. 325–334, or Israel, 2004, pp. 191–261), a major incentive to revise some of the standard approaches stems from the historiographical problem of emigration-induced change, which has been researched from multiple perspectives in the humanities and social sciences. Not only did scholars draw on individual and collective biographies but they also measured "substantial impact parameters," using bibliometric methods, membership issues in academic associations, and statistics regarding the leading positions in scholarly societies, which were particularly applied to the "hard sciences," such as physics and chemistry, as well as sociology and political science in the "soft sciences" (Juette, 1990; Soellner, 1996).

The impulses for such a revised research strategy came from relatively new approaches to the historiography of the cultural context of science (Galison, Graubard, & Mendelsohn, 2001; Schmidgen, Geimer, & Dierig, 2004; Erikson, 2005) and problems of the transfer of knowledge (Argote, 1999; Jankrift & Steger, 2004; Ash & Soellner, 2006). In applying those new perspectives to the research networks and the communication structures of émigré neuroscientists, this article aims to provide additional perspectives towards the social background and cultural implications of the case of forced migration in the neuroscience field (cf. Peiffer, 1998a, 1998b, 1998c). An earlier process-oriented perspective developed in the 1990s by a group of scholars at the *Berliner Wissenschaftskolleg* has opened promising paths for the study "of [the] intellectual and cultural change" occurring through the forced migration of European scientific émigrés (Ash & Soellner, 1996, pp. 1–19). A number of American and German historians and philosophers of science (Fischer, 1996) have provided useful models through their scholarship on emigration-induced scientific change. These included the relevant social accounts of the historical developments, social reception, and reintegration of German-speaking émigré scientists. As such, refugee-neuroscientists, like all their compatriots in exile, found themselves in the foreign environment of North America, where they had to continue their daily life, support their partners and families, become relicensed and obtain professional acceptance. They had to learn the social and cultural codes, psychological mentality, and likewise "soft working skills" often the "hard way" (Rheinberger, 2005, pp. 187–197) when being barred from clinical work, having to close labs in order to pursue better paid jobs for their subsistence, or changing their personal research interests so as to "fit" more closely with the acceptable clinical and scientific paradigms of the often hands-on, capitalist, and technophile North American society.

From neuropathology to psychoanalytic psychiatry and medical education: The case example of Karl Stern

Many of the émigré neuroscientists, just to name the neuropathologist Karl Stern (1906–1975), and his colleagues from the former group of Kurt Goldstein (1878–1965), Adhémar Gelb (1887–1936), Victor Franz (1883–1950), and Walther Riese (1890–1976) in Frankfurt am Main, were influenced by interpretations of holistic neurology and the experimental culture of the Weimar Period, which they at first sought to continue in their American exile (Stahnisch & Pow, 2015). What emanates as the central problem for émigré neuroscientists such as Stern and Goldstein, was not only personal acculturation but also the readjustment of their research and clinical activities. They had to search for new work places and integration into the preexisting Canadian and US working groups, research programs, and academic milieus, which they often literally encountered as a "New World." Continuous comparisons of the similarities and differences with their former European experiences were permanently present (Sachs, 1998), a process through which they noticeably stood out due to their critique and reproaches of the differences, shortfalls, and exaggerations of life in their new host countries. For example, the Goldstein collaborator from Berlin Max Bielschowsky (1869–1940) wrote back from his own exile abroad:

> I am as well as a man with my past could be in a very strange country [*auf fremdem Boden*]. You know how much I love my home country [*meine Heimat*]. All the friendliness and kind offers of support by my [new] colleagues, however, will never really substitute for what I had to leave behind [in Germany].[1]

The members of the Goldstein Group certainly proved to be no exception to that rule, no matter what their influential contributions to neurology, psychiatry, experimental psychology, or matters of the philosophy of science and medicine had been. This loose network of people included the earlier collaborators from Frankfurt am Main and

---

[1] Émigré neurohistologist Max Bielschowsky, *Letter*, qtd. after Peiffer (2004), p. 496.

Berlin, Karl Stern who had joined the Allan Memorial Institute of psychiatric research at McGill University in Montreal, Canada), Walther Riese who immigrated to Richmond, Virginia, in the United States, Frieda Fromm-Reichmann (1889–1957) who received a position as a psychiatrist at the Chestnut Lodge mental asylum in Maryland in the United States and who independently immigrated to other destinations in North America. Goldstein's nearest friend and colleague Adhémar Gelb (1887–1936) had lost his chair at the University of Halle and was just about to leave Germany in 1936 for a position at Kansas State University in Manhattan, Kansas, when he succumbed, at the age of 49, to a tuberculosis infection, which he had contracted in his continuous work with severe clinical patients (Danzer, 2006, p. 23f).

The case of Goldstein's collaborator Stern in Montreal, a former pupil of brain oncologist Walther Spielmeyer (1879–1935) in Munich, can be presented here as an important change from an accomplished neuropathologist back in Germany, who later became a well-accepted clinical psychiatrist and fervent academic teacher later in Canada. At first glance, the conditions for a transfer of concepts and methods were ideal in Stern's case (Goldblatt, 1992, pp. 279–282), who was born in a small town in Bavaria near the Czech border (Bullemer, 2003).[2] After he had passed most of his medical education at the Charité Hospital and Medical School in Berlin, Stern graduated with an MD in 1930 from the University of Frankfurt/M. Between 1930 and 1931, he worked together with Goldstein as a resident physician in psychiatry at the Frankfurt Neurological Institute (Stahnisch, 2008).

Between 1932 and 1933, he had a Rockefeller fellowship in the Department of Neuropathology at the German Research Institute for Psychiatry (Deutsche Forschungsanstalt fuer Psychiatrie: DFA) in Munich to collaborate with the neurohistologist Spielmeyer, one of the world-leading specialists at the time for brain-tumor diagnoses which provided the basis for fruitful scientific publications (Stern, 1939). Here, he had procured a position, in which, apart from the pathological analysis of the brains in "idiocy" and "circulatory disturbances," he mainly acted as Spielmeyer's teaching assistant. Yet, this implied an enormous effort to live up to the high standards of Spielmeyer's expertise in this area. (This is all the more crucial, as one of the members of the leading Spanish school — Rafael Lorente de No [1902–1990] and Pío del Rio Hortega [1882–1945] and Oskar [1870–1959] and Cécile Vogt [1875–1962] in Berlin—worked on the same scientific level worldwide.) He was also expected to introduce graduate students and visiting researchers into the various histological methods and the vast array of laboratory applications in use by Spielmeyer so that for a large part of the day, Stern had "to wander from microscope to microscope in order to instruct the guests" (Stern, 1951, p. 16). In Munich, Stern clearly worked at the cutting-edge of neuroscience research and medical education at large.

When Goldstein decided to leave Frankfurt am Main in 1930 for Berlin (Kreft, 1997, pp. 131–144), he asked Stern to join him again as a consultant in one of his psychiatry wards. Since Stern had by that time received a great reputation for being a proficient neurohistologist himself, he was also expected to do the brain autopsies in the Moabit *Prosectur*. It seems that Stern, with his broad interests and knowledge basis, squared very well with Goldstein's holistic neurological assumptions which integrated philosophy, social psychiatry, and neuroscientific innovations alike. Concerned with medical processes

---

[2]The village of Cham has now named a "Dr.-Karl-Stern-Straße" in his honor and has commemorated his expulsion from Germany.

of adaptation and healing, rather than with aggressive "extinction," holist neurology sat at the center of what Nazi ideology later rejected as "weak" Jewish medicine, while Stern himself did not hesitate at all to follow his mentor to the German Capital:

> The hours were from six to eight but frequently we worked until well after midnight. There I found myself in a strange and extraordinary world, entirely different from anything I have ever seen before. We saw a continuous stream of clients. There were mothers with children who had just left a home destroyed by an alcoholic. These were drunkards, morphine and cocaine addicts, the hopeless, the destitute, those who had cynically and rebelliously isolated themselves, bound to a life of increasing solitude and destruction, and those who had succumbed to the deficiency of a loveless world. This was a cross-section through the darkest layer of the city. It was that fringe of life where human existence is ultimately atomized and surrounds itself with a void, a space of negation. It would take a whole book to describe all this so that the reader would be able to re-experience it. [...] I never recovered from these experiences. That means that I never recovered the undergraduate's boundless admiration for science and for the absolute sacredness of research. [...] Although I had more scientific training later, I never forget those experiences in Moabit. They seemed to have put the abstract scientific aspect of Medicine into its proper place. It is just one side of a profound and complex development that with many of us science and art in medicine are no longer integrated. As science in general, medical science has gained in extensiveness what it has lost in intensity. (Stern, 1951, p. 85f)

Moabit was then one of the few academic hospitals with different services in neurology, psychiatry, and pathology that similarly related to each other as in the huge Neurological Institute, which Goldstein directed in Frankfurt before. However, just as everything was set for Goldstein's clinic to develop into one of the major centers of German neurology, the catastrophe began. As soon as the Nazis had seized power, Goldstein was incarcerated and only released after agreeing to leave Germany forever. Through Switzerland, where he cofounded the "Emergency Society for German Scholars in Exile" ("*Notgemeinschaft Deutscher Wissenschaftler im Ausland*") together with the Budapest pathologist Philip Schwarz (1894–1962) and the Mainz novelist Carl Zuckmayer (1896–1977), he sought refuge in Amsterdam, finishing his seminal publication *DerAufbau des Organismus* [The Architecture of the Organism] (Harrington, 1991, pp. 299–304).

Stern stayed in Germany until 1935, before he left for London and eventually reached New York. Here a tight networking between contemporary international scientists comes into play, as his mentor from Munich days, Walther Spielmeyer, had met the Montreal neurosurgeon Wilder Penfield (1891–1976), previously familiar with Stern's work, on Penfield's lecture tour to North and South America in 1931 (Weber, 2000, p. 240f). Also, Stern's new acquaintance with "a Canadian neurophysiologist" at Queen Square — who had supposedly been Herbert H. Hyland (1900–1977) from Toronto and who was in London exactly during this time — helped likewise so that Stern could leave for Montreal, where he immediately began to work in a mental hospital then on the outskirts of the city ("*Hôspital de Nôtre Dame*").[3] As Penfield was to inaugurate a psychiatric department to complete his Neurological Institute, he recommended Stern

---

[3]Spielmeyer had already gotten in contact with Penfield through letter communication by Otfrid Foerster (1873–1941). He was later invited by the Montreal neurosurgeon to visit the Neurological Institute of McGill University on his lecture tour to North America. Also a transatlantic contact endured between Goldstein and Franz Alexander (1891–1964), since both had frequently been encountered at the joint seminars of the Neurological Institute with the Psychoanalytical Institute in Frankfurt am Main (see Laier, 1994, pp. 176–186).

to the biological psychiatrist D. Ewen Cameron (1901–1967) as the designated director. Shortly after the Allan Memorial Institute (AMI) had opened, in 1943, Stern was explicitly working for the latter's Geriatric Unit together with the Czech-born and German-trained physician Vojtech Albert Kral (1903–1988) (see Fig. 1). He further taught the students' courses as a research assistant, and later as an assistant professor for psychiatry (Hogan, 2007, pp. 131–150). However, as Stern admits in his autobiography *The Pillar of Fire*, his interests in neuro-oncology and the cognitive defects in clinical psychiatry went further than the narrow program, as well as the the routine culture at the Montreal Neurological Institute (MNI) and the Royal Victoria Hospital. In fact, Stern came into a preexisting interdisciplinary hospital setting, which was soon conceptually and also locally separated between its main players, the MNI and AMI. The MNI mainly fulfilled Penfield's specific needs, that is, the different departments of epileptology, neurosurgery, neurology, and neuropathology were service institutions for an extended research program for the mapping of the human cortex. Not regarding the personally problematic relationship between renowned Professor Cameron, and the émigré psychiatrist Stern on his staff, Stern also left Montreal at the end of the 1950s to assume a leading role in clinical psychiatry in Ottawa. Between 1951 and 1975, he continued to work as a clinical psychiatrist at the University of Ottawa, yet no longer being a laboratory brain researcher. For more than a decade, he also served as the head

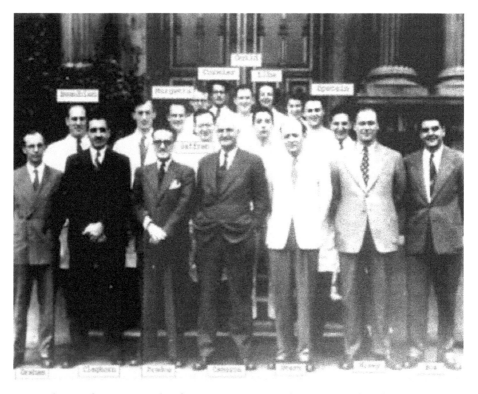

Figure 1. Karl Stern (first person right of D. Ewan Cameron in the center) at the Allan Memorial Institute (AMI), circa 1946. © Dr. Theodore I. Sourkes, McGill University, Montreal, Canada. Reproduced by permission of Dr. Theodore I. Sourkes, McGill University, Montreal, Canada. Permission to reuse must be obtained from the rightsholder.

of the psychiatry department and promoted an integrative clinical approach that also encompassed psychoanalytical therapy options (Stahnisch & Pow, 2015, p. 246).

At first glance, conditions for the transfer of ideas and methods were ideal in the case of Karl Stern, although his biography cannot really be regarded as a success story in terms of theory change in the neurosciences. On the one hand, Goldstein's group, to which he belonged in the early 1930s, was about to transfer Moabit Hospital into one of the country's major centers for neuroscientific research, but the *Machtergreifung* of the Nazis diminished all their plans. It represents in a nutshell many other areas of medical science that stood in opposition to the ideals of Nazism and could not continue as traditions in Germany. With a view to the cultural picture of science, holist neurology ceased to exist, when the Goldstein group continued its work in spheres of clinical and experimental psychology. On the other hand, Stern himself came into a preexisting interdisciplinary hospital setting at the MNI, which was highly organized, although not in a broad and holistic fashion as many German centers. It rather fulfilled Penfield's and later Cameron's specific research needs (Feindel, 1991, p. 821f).

This story is far from complete, however, if it is not considered in terms of personal success and institutional change. Numerous oral history accounts underline Stern's noteworthy talent as an academic teacher, who seemed to have interested a whole new generation of Montreal medical students in the histological study of the brain (Feindel, 1984, pp. 347–358). It also informs us about the necessity of broad education and training, often forgotten by a disciplinary tunnel vision on scientific excellence dis-respecting a solid training base as the source for future innovations. The view on the cultural picture of science thus shows that Stern's life and work was doubly prevented from blossoming into a full biomedical career — in the beginning years by National Socialist-politics and then as a coworker to Cameron's program. His case can thus be seen as a "conversion" from a basic neuroscientific researcher into a fervent clinician and influential university teacher. Thus, Stern's case counts in favor of the assumption that emigration-induced scientific change must be separated from general scientific change at various levels from the individual to the cultural, although in this example this would have to be done in a narrow if not to say "negative" sense. In contrast with the first example and despite the emigration of a mind with its methods, no thorough induction of scientific change can be identified in Stern's case, but contrafactually might have well been, if the facilities at Moabit Hospital had not been resolved by Nazi officials.

Similar to Stern's individual fate in Canada, the Goldstein group fell apart and the research of its members took on a very different direction. Goldstein himself entered a private practice of neurology and psychiatry, after he had arrived in New York City in 1935, dispersing his own work between an appointment as clinical teacher of psychopathology at Columbia and further running a small neurophysiological laboratory at Montefiore Hospital.[4] Although he stayed in close letter exchanges with other diaspora members of this former group, they all now went their own ways, such as the neuropathologist Walther Riese (Stahnisch & Pow, 2014, pp. 2466–2468), who now worked at the Medical College in Richmond, Virginia. Riese also left holist neurology and ventured into theoretical neuropsychology, and later medical history. Goldstein's former clinical psychologist, Adhémar Gelb, had died in 1936, after losing his

---

[4]See also Holdorff (2016) in this special issue.

chair at the University of Halle and not living up to travel to the United States, where he was to assume a professorship in experimental psychology offered to him by Kansas University. The decline of the school was further reflected in Stern's fate in Canada, who rather supplemented the neuropathological expertise at Montreal's MNI and AMI, before deciding to continue his work later as a clinical psychiatrist in Ottawa.[5]

With a view to the cultural perspective of scientific and clinical practice, it is certainly possible to see the cases of Stern, Goldstein, and Riese not simply as additional biographies related to the forced migration wave from Germany. Instead, their histories tell us more about the actual production processes of knowledge in medicine and neuroscience. On the one hand, Goldstein's group was clearly about to transfer Moabit Hospital into an important center for neuroscientific research in Germany, but the *Machtergreifung* of the Nazis diminished all their plans. On the other hand, all of these émigré neuroscientists came into preexisting clinical and research settings with their specific interplay of conceptual, personal, and research relations, in which, taking up a word of Stern's (1951, p. 77), "methods [had already] become mentalities." That is, they had to cope with the local North American research cultures and mostly had to abandon their own holistic ideas to more applied forms of neurology and patient testing, however, still influencing local practices: In Stern's case, a strong emphasis on psychoanalytical psychopathology, in Goldstein's example, a thorough way of clinical observation and history taking, and Riese served as an important role model in his faculty, combining in-depth neuropathological knowledge with clinical alertness and a wide range of historical and interdisciplinary scholarship. So in their local settings, there still survived a bit of "holist patina," which impressed faculty colleagues and strongly influenced their students. And Stern was also very influential in his relation to the younger faculty members at the AMI, for example, as the later psychiatrist and psycho-immunologist Dr. Edrita Fried (b. 1934), associate in Stern's service, has stated (Sourkes & Pinard, 1995, p. 151).

The instances of "scientific" and "knowledge changes" that can be extracted from this case example both apply to laboratory and clinical practice as well as to the emergence of new kinds of interdisciplinarity: The reconstruction of differing neuroscientific research styles or cultures hence shows the necessity to go beyond the more "classical" perspectives of the history of ideas, of institutional historiography, or the writing of individual scientists' biographies and to take the communication and teaching networks of the émigrés into account as well. This holds for the cultural patterns inscribed into thought and practice, national identities, and international contacts during the constitutional phase of the emerging neurosciences (Rosen, 1944, p. 39).[6] Thus, it becomes possible to study the interdisciplinary exchanges in a rather in-depth manner as these continued in both collaborative clinical and theoretical work despite the disrupted and dispersed local contexts along the American East Coast, mediated by letter exchanges, phone calls, and the still very dense railway system in the 1950s.

---

[5]University Archives of the University of Ottawa, ON (Fonds 43 NB-3056, Karl Stern, Human Resources Files; Fonds 6 NB-9656.8), *passim*.

[6]The role of "the stranger" in creating innovative fields and disciplines in new cultural environments is of pivotal importance. Just as the social need for comparison in the immigrant individual becomes a vital property for adaptation in the new cultural surrounding, the ability to criticize and relate to preexisting research traditions assumes ample input from local cultural values, readily shaped interpretations of new observations, or clinical skills. An important, though quite dated source in related medical historiography is Rosen (1944, p. 39).

From clinical neurology and psychiatry to public mental health: The case example of Robert Weil

With respect to the North American medical context in the 1930s, and apart from the philanthropic endeavors of the "Emergency Committee for Displaced Physicians" (Zimmerman, 2006), and the assumed responsibility of the Rockefeller Foundation for its former fellows and awardees, there had to be either a substantial need for research expansion or some perceived deficiency in scientific competences and clinical care, before the knowledge of the émigrés could come into play (Pearle, 1984). Until that was the case and even in times of the transition into émigrés' resumption of professional work, they relied heavily on scientific colleagues, politicians, business men, and even family members to facilitate their reintegration process in their new host countries. In fact, landing in the United States outside of the contemporary population quotas for German, Austrian, Czech, and Polish immigrants or without sufficient proof of having been a university teacher in the country of origin was only possible through the individual affidavit of American citizens who declared to sustain émigrés in times of financial hardship (Davie & Koenig, 1949, pp. 160–162).

Beyond émigrés' positive experiences, the failures, backlashes, and even hostilities that many of the émigrés neuroscientists had to face in their private and working lives, deserve further scrutiny. This was particularly the case during the early years following their arrival in a generally anti-German and often even outright anti-Semitic climate before the war, which led to their exclusion from the professional job market, cultural misunderstandings as to their former positions, along with insufficient language proficiency that created many disturbances among their academic peers (Stortz, 2003, pp. 231–235). In addition, there was also a widespread mood of resignation among many of the German-speaking émigrés, particularly during the first three years of the war, when the *Blitzkrieg* brought many European countries under Nazi occupation and when family members had been imprisoned or even interned in penitentiaries and concentration camps. For some, they simply had not received any news from their loved ones on the other side of the Atlantic. Like many other contemporary immigrant groups, German-speaking émigrés also used to stay together in similar neighborhoods of major North American cities, such as the Lower East Side in New York City, Clayton Neighborhood of St. Louis, or Pacific Palisades near Los Angeles. Their constant devaluations of American culture were proverbial, with ongoing exchanges about their former experiences from previous lives in Central Europe. In their *Kaffeekraentzchen*, Salons, and *Gespraechsrunden*, which often became known as the group meetings of the Beiunskys ("*bien de chez nous*") (Sachs, 1998), there was no separation by profession between scientists, artists, and writers, of course, serving the basic functions for moral and practical support in continued interdisciplinary exchanges (Grob, 1983).

By applying a network-oriented approach to such historical processes, the "classical" perspectives confined to certain types of "gains" and "losses" in differing neuroscientific research styles is decisively widened. Such a network approach may indeed be seen as a reformulation of what Harvard historian of science Thomas S. Kuhn (1922–1996) had once called a "disciplinary matrix" (Kuhn, 1977), that is, the commitment and involvement of individual scientists to the shared conceptual resources, values, instruments, techniques, and practices of their respective community. Thus, in the field of the neurosciences, the actions of the main players and mediators of such a matrix may be feasibly reconstructed with regard to varying organizational and contextual points (Meyer, 2001, p. 93). Regarding such specific scholarly networks in relation to others, it has to be born in mind that their forms and characteristics varied markedly due to their intrinsic composition through the academics, economists, politicians, and non-professional actors involved. However, their results may in the end be quite equivalent, as most academic, clinical, or organizational positions were acquired via personal relations, academic references, and the reputation of the teaching or research institutions at the time. This leads also back to the central question on the elements that have triggered and fostered the theory-change in the neurosciences under various cultural, social, and institutional conditions. Exemplary are the official as well as unofficial networks within the German Research Society, the Kaiser–Wilhelm Society, and the early German Research Institution for Psychiatry that played major roles in the support, placement, and connection of the émigré neuroscientists from Central Europe in the United States and Canada (Hammerstein, 2000, pp. 219–224). Here, it is important to methodologically integrate the status of collective biographies, scientific networks, and interdisciplinary endeavors into this particular historical analysis of knowledge change in the neurosciences. In this respect, it will have to be kept in mind that not only highly skilled individual researchers had to leave Central European universities during the Nazi period, but also often whole research schools were forcefully expelled from the German-speaking countries.

As an example, I want to draw the attention to the case of clinical neurologist and psychiatrist Robert Weil (see Fig. 2), who belonged to a group of German-educated

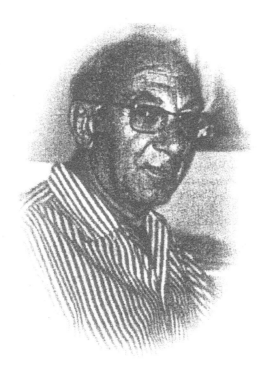

Figure 2. Robert Weil from the program invitation to his funeral ceremony in 2002 (Robert Weil Correspondence, MS-2-750, 2003-047, Box 5, File 1). Courtesy of the Robert Weil fonds (MS-10-1), Dalhousie University Archives, Halifax, Nova Scotia.

neuroscientists of the provinces of the former Austrian-Hungarian Double-Monarchy. He was born into a Jewish family in a rural part of Bohemia, yet in his adolescence he converted to Lutheran Protestantism. Weil was one of many clinical and social psychiatrists during the 1930s, who displayed a profound research interest in various areas of psychiatry, ranging from nosology, psychoanalysis well over to the neuro- and histopathology of the brain. He had graduated from the German University of Prague in 1933 and pursued postgraduate studies in neurology and psychiatry at the Vienna Medical School. He then worked as an Army psychiatrist between 1935 and 1938 in Prague and in Bohemia, before he fled together with his family for the United Kingdom and later to Canada, following the annexation and the ceding of parts of Czechoslovakia to Germany (Baglole, 2002, p. 64). With many other émigré medical scientists, after the passage to Canada, Weil shared the fate of many émigrés of being transported to one of the more remote areas of Saskatchewan in the Prairies, where he was allowed to practice medicine as a general practitioner between the years of 1939 and 1942. Until 1944 he interned in neurosurgery at the Saskatoon City Hospital and eventually during the war years, Weil managed to work with the Saskatchewan Mental Health Service until 1949. This marked a time of psychiatric care that he saw as "predominantly practiced under poor conditions in mental Hospitals," and in which he regarded university psychiatric teaching to be "uncommon as a subject of study in Canadian Universities."[7] In comparison, neurology and psychiatry at the Charles University of Prague — Weil's alma mater — had previously risen to international recognition under Arnold Pick (1851–1924) and Ladislav Haškovec (1866–1944), who expanded compulsory university training in neuropsychiatry, psycho-pathology, and areas of social psychiatry to all medical graduates.

Consequently, in this institution and later by his colleagues of the Saskatchewan Mental Hospital at Battleford, it was realized that Weil was a broadly trained psychiatrist and neurologist, who had a lot of experiences in field psychiatry, due to his earlier appointment in the medical service of the Czech Army. His biography thus represents one of numerous examples, in which a neuroscientist arriving from Central-Europe found poor clinical and mental health conditions in North America in comparison with those he was acquainted with in the German-speaking context.[8] As Weil perceived it, the subject of mental health was quite

---

[7]Letter of Robert Weil, Halifax, NS, to the psychiatrist Dr. Charles A. Roberts (1918–1996) in Ottawa, dating June-7, 1986: "In 1942 I joined the Mental Health Services of Saskatchewan, my first position [in Canada] being a junior psychiatrist in the Sask. Mental Hospital in Battleford. The medical superintendent at that time was Dr. J[ack]. J. McNeil [b. 1918]—a native of Summerside, P.E.I. Dr. McNeil was a great friend of Dr. Clarence [M.] Hincks [1885–1965] who visited our hospital almost yearly. On one of these visits he was accompanied by Dr. J. Griffin. Both sat in on our conferences and also gave us the opportunity to meet and get to know them in personal conversations. Both Clarence and Jack were always welcommed [!] [sic] visitors who brought us all kind of informations [!] [sic] about the psychiatric activities, developments etc from all the provinces. They also shared with us their visions and plans for the improvements in the care for the mentally ill."; citation taken from his typographed letter – from the folders on the Robert Weil Correspondence (Ms 2-750, Call # 2003-47, Box 8, File 15, p. 1) in the Dalhousie University Archives & Special Collections, Killam Memorial Library, Halifax, NS.

[8]For Weil's perception of the Canadian context of psychiatry and mental health see "Group for the Advancement of Psychiatry. Reports"; "Notes & Articles on 'Interdisciplinary Research' "; materials from the folders of the Robert Weil Collection (Ms 2-750, Call # 2003-47, Accession Report, Box 2, File 5; Box 5, File 3) in the Dalhousie University Archives & Special Collections, Killam Memorial Library, Halifax, NS.

uncommon at Canadian Universities and not very well established as a serviceable system in the rural areas of the country. At this critical juncture of his career, his broad knowledge in psychiatry, his engagement in setting up a wider Mental Health system, and his social contacts with leading members of the Saskatchewan Health Service and the Canadian psychiatric community earned him such recognition that Weil was hired as the first assistant Professor of Psychiatry by Dalhousie University in Nova Scotia. He even managed to get this post against the stern reluctance of the Officers of the Medical Society of Nova Scotia and their earlier policy, lasting between 1910 and 1930, not to accept "aliens" and "Jewish-born doctors" from other countries (Hincks, 1947, pp. 161–165). Weil stayed at Dalhousie University from 1950 to 1975 and then retired at the level of an associate professor. As a member of its core faculty, he exerted a strong influence on the hiring policy of that university and the organizational restructuring of its services in psychiatry, neurology, and neuropathology, in which he promoted a "German" educational style of general knowledge in psychiatric training. It is remarkable, and yet typical of many other émigré neuroscientists, that Weil displayed a thoroughly "scientist attitude" to a variety of perspectives on psychiatry. Although strongly influenced by experiencing his and his wife's expulsion from their home country as well as the general political events, which he academically discussed and heavily criticized in many of his papers and articles. He believed in a unifying and quite cathartic effect of science on its digression in ideology and technocracy. In a way, a general outlook of science and the humanist attitude in psychiatry served for him as *residuum non destructum* in times of personal despair and general political worries after his immigration to Canada:

> This discrepancy between our knowledge and our behavior makes it so difficult today to orient oneself in this chaos of our enigmatic world. Man now stands confused before his own creation complicated by so many technical devices which he is unable to control. And in his confusion and his insecurity he is always more tempted to reach for a gun than for an instrument of peace. War appears to be still a better and safer alternative to a peaceful adjustment of our environment to our needs and a better adaptation of mankind to the material world which presents itself to us.
>
> As you see, there are two main problems we have to face in modern time. Firstly, we have to utilize our knowledge for practical application — that is a matter of economics and politics and therefore outside of my realm.
>
> The second large problem of mankind is a psychological one. It is the problem of the adjustment of individuals and groups to the environment which is set for him the moment he is born. It is also the problem of redirecting our mental potentialities to a healthier attitude towards the material world which surrounds us & towards our fellowmen.[9]

Weil was also one of the founding members of the "Canadian Psychiatric Association" (CPA) and later in 1968 also its president. His work thoroughly introduced German ideas of social psychiatry and interdisciplinary teaching and research, while helping to establish a more effective level of education and patient care in the Canadian public mental health system (Dowbiggin, 2003). His stronger engagement with mental health issues can be seen as an individual example of change from his primary interest in somatic neurology and neuropathology. Neither in the Czech army nor in the Canadian health system could his interests be fully met (Dalhousie University, 2002, p. 1). What this example shows,

---

[9] From Weil's address to the CPA in 1953; citation taken from his manuscript – Typography from the folders on the Robert Weil Correspondence (Ms 2-750, Call # 2003-47, Box 6, File 15) in the Dalhousie University Archives & Special Collections, Killam Memorial Library, Halifax, NS.

however, is definitely not that Canadian social psychiatry and the development of Dalhousie's facilities in the neurosciences could not have emerged without Robert Weil. It makes plausible that under his supervision and tutelage, the historical course taken would have had a different velocity and would have ventured into new directions (Weil & Demay, 1947; Weil, 1960). The course of these events certainly appears to be a mixture of institutional circumstances and biographical factors, as this highly intellectual man, who not only reflected in numerous sociological and philosophical articles on the cultural background of the neurosciences but also shaped and reshaped the research outlook of areas of biological psychiatry and bench neuroscience at his university, proved himself to be an effective and pragmatic science organizer, who integrated these ideas into the institutional setting of his medical school. Dalhousie, at that time, experienced an increase from two to eight professorships in neurology, psychiatry, neuropathology, and neuroanatomy, while he was an active faculty member.[10]

The central points addressed by Weil also strongly influenced a development in Canada, which Gerald Grob has characterized as "the emphasis on the prevention and on the provision of care and treatment in the community" for US psychiatry (Grob, 1983, p. 232). The mental health problem from large hospitalization numbers was perceived as highly demanding also by the psychiatrists of the Canadian and American psychiatric clinics and asylums — thus bearing widespread implications for the mental health system. It is important to see that émigré doctors exerted a strong impact on the Canadian and US mental health systems, which was, however, preceded by reevaluations going on in various parts of Europe, mainly in areas of the former Austro-Hungarian Empire, in Italy, Switzerland, and Germany.

From brain psychiatry to clinical neurochemistry: The case example of Heinz Lehmann

These particular refugee scientists and medical doctors must have been well trained to arrive at a tenacity of solving problems and overcoming all sorts of constraints and obstacles in their clinical or laboratory research, as was the case with many émigré neuroscientists, who had been trained in some of the leading centers in Central Europe. From a social history viewpoint, the emigration of scientists and scholars after 1933 can even be understood as a spectacular case of forced international elite-circulation, but that circulation did not happen automatically. Instead, before we may take scientific change into account, we need to question who got the opportunity to continue or begin scientific work, and thus at least a potential position to participate in changes of research trends in his or her host country? Very likely, those individuals had to have the necessary aptitude to convince greater audiences, as well as the social and basic linguistic competences to negotiate budgets with administrative officers. That the requirement of such "soft skills" is far from trivial would become fairly obvious in the case of many émigré neuroscientists, who often needed to pass medical exams before being allowed to practice again. They had

---

[10]"Dalhousie University. Faculty of Medicine. Committee on medical Education. Elective Programme"; materials from the folders of the Robert Weil Collection (Ms 2-750, Call # 2003-47, Accession Report, 1st p., Box 5, File 3; Box 6, File 11) in the Dalhousie University Archives & Special Collections, Killam Memorial Library, Halifax, NS.

to find jobs in research institutes or medical faculties, and were to serve in low-paid or nonsalaried "voluntary" positions, etc. (Grossman, 1993).

For example, other "research import products" from émigré neurologists and psychiatrists — such as the neurorehabilitative approach of the holist neurologist Kurt Goldstein from Frankfurt and Berlin, the psychiatric genetics and epidemiology of the Berlin psychiatrist Franz Josef Kallmann (1897–1965), or the introduction of the psychopharmacological Chlorpromazine therapy[11]—for a long time stood in the cultural shadow of dominant psychoanalytical theories. In American psychiatry, the clinical psychoanalysts influenced both the state hospital system as well as the large psychiatric hospitals of the Veterans Administration between the 1940s and the 1960s, before these major approaches further developed into some important research traditions in the field of modern neuroscience.[12] Moreover, Heinz Lehmann at the Allan Memorial Institute, the psychiatry department at McGill, contributed the first research publications on chlorpromazine in English in 1953 and, three years later, on the antidepressant imipramine (Anonymous, 1993, pp. 141f). Lehmann represented one of those German-speaking émigré physicians with whom Weil upheld continuous letter exchanges after their mutual emigration to Canada.[13]

When looking more closely at the contributions of individual émigré neuroscientists, such as Heinz Lehmann at McGill University, the role and influence of the process of reintegration of the exiled neuroscientists in Canada and the United States becomes more comprehensible. The vital function served by North America was that of a safe haven for the expelled scientists and intellectuals, a harbor for ideas, epistemologies, and innovative experiments, and a refuge for Europe's cast-off intelligentsia during the rise of the Nazi tyranny, Holocaust, and Second World War. Despite a certain amount of attention paid to these "homeless intellectuals" in recent publications (Weindling, 1989; Deichmann, 1996; Israel, 2004), their impact on and relation to American science and medical culture has not yet been fully explored. For many, coming to North America was like:

> parachuting from Europe into the new world of North American psychiatry at the very brink of WWII with nothing in my backpack other than Kraepelin's and Bleuler's guides to the diagnosis of the major psychoses, manic-depressive disorder, and schizophrenia. We had only two theories to explain the rest of the psychiatric illnesses, the neuroses and personality disorders: Freud's psychoanalysis and Pavlov's and Skinner's findings on conditioning and learning.[14]

---

[11]Chlorpromazine therapy had been introduced by the psychiatrist and biochemist Heinz Lehmann, who had promoted the development in the French-speaking literature also among the English-speaking North American research communities in psychiatry and neurology.

[12]Personal interview with MNI neurologist Fred Andermann, May 26, 2007, in the Faculty Club of McGill University in Montreal, PQ.

[13]For example, letter on August 19, 1953 by Robert Weil to Heinz Edgar Lehmann about the issue of clinical hypnosis and their mutual work on the Canadian Special Commission on "Hypnosis" and "Hypnoanalysis." Materials from the folders of the Robert Weil Collection (Ms 2-750, Call # 2003-47, Accession Report, Box 2, File 5; Box 5, File 3) in the Dalhousie University Archives.

[14]Heinz Lehmann, 1995. Autographical Papers. Personal File (Professor H. Lehmann), Collections of the University Archives, McGill University, Montreal, Canada.

Faced not only with expulsion from academic working circles but also prohibited from pursuing their career (a "*Berufsverbot*"), many of the neuroscientists looked at, here, searched to escape the situation in the German-speaking countries and to establish a new professional life elsewhere.

This was also the case in the clinical neurologist and psychiatrist Lehmann, who had been born as the son of a Jewish physician in Berlin (see Fig. 3). He had himself studied medicine in Marburg, as well as at the psychiatric centers of Freiburg in Germany and Vienna in Austria. Between 1935 and 1937, he pursued postgraduate research while being a staff-attending physician ("*Assistenzarzt*") at the Martin Luther Stift and at the Jewish hospital of Berlin. In 1937, after he had been barred to continue his medical work as a hospital physician even for his Jewish patients, he managed to immigrate to Canada on a tourist visa. Immediately after his arrival in Montreal in Quebec, he was offered the position of a hospital physician at the Verdun Protestant Hospital, which became the main clinical center of the psychiatric research divisions of McGill University's Allan Memorial Institute (AMI). Rising fast through the academic ranks, in 1947, he even became its clinical chief, which was rather a parallel reflection of the research interests of the somatic psychiatrist Cameron at the AMI. Yet, other than in the example of Karl Stern, Lehmann could benefit strongly from the support of the scientific and clinical milieu of the AMI with its contemporary biological research

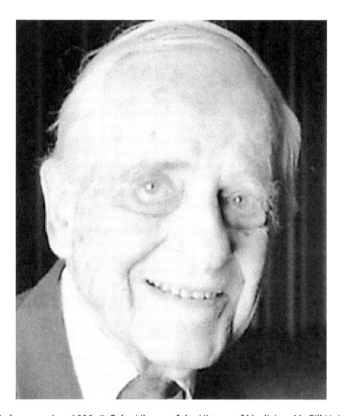

Figure 3. Heinz Lehmann, circa 1990. © Osler Library of the History of Medicine, McGill University, Montreal, Quebec, Canada. Reproduced by permission of the Osler Library of the History of Medicine, McGill University, Montreal, Quebec, Canada. Permission to reuse must be obtained from the rightsholder.

programs (Sourkes & Pinard, 1995, pp. 10–15). At the same time, Lehmann managed to turn his solid education in French language from his Berlin high school times into a large medical asset (Lehmann, 1983, pp. 145–154). Shortly after chlorpromazine had been developed by the psychiatrists and neurochemists, Jean Delay (1907–1987) and Pierre Deniker (1917–1998) in France in 1952 after World War II, Lehmann introduced the drug among the English-speaking clinical neuroscientists in North America. Lehmann now redirected his own psychiatric research solely from a psychopharmaceutical perspective and particularly towards the treatment of schizophrenic patients. One could even go so far as to view his work at McGill University as a stepping stone for his additional activities in psychiatry and public mental health in the provincial Comité de la Santé Mentale de Quebéc, as an American Fellow of the Collegium Internationale Neuro-Psychopharmacologium, along with being a Canadian representative and expert for the World Health Organization in New York.

A defining feature for the biographical differences between Stern and Lehmann had openly been their diverging socialization in the medical research landscape in Germany before their forced migration to Canada. Of course, they both had excellent language proficiency in French, which they could further perfect while working in the French-Canadian surroundings of Montreal. However, both émigré neuroscientists used these soft skills in quite different ways: While Stern primarily related to the francophone scientific community of Quebec and aligned through his scientific connections particularly with the psychoanalytically schooled psychiatrists of France and Quebec, Lehmann emerged as a decisive bridge-builder between the new biological tradition of psychopharmacology in France and French-speaking Switzerland with their developed pharmaceutical and chemical industries. Lehmann was an important gatekeeper, who could introduce these impulses and initiatives into the English-speaking world of North American psychiatry (Stip, 2015, p. S5).

Another instructive example of a successful, though slightly changing career in the clinical neurosciences, is the professional Silberberg-couple from Breslau, where the female pathologist Ruth Silberberg (1906–1997) had to work four years without salary while her husband, the neurohistologist Martin Silberberg (1895–1969), had to change from one low-paid and short-term position to the next one, first working in Halifax, Nova Scotia, in Canada, then in New York City and St. Louis in the United States. In his letter exchange with his mentor, the American physician Leo Loeb (1869–1959), Martin Silberberg respectively wrote on August 4, 1938, on the occasion of a job opening at the Middlesex University in Massachusetts:

> Dear Dr. Loeb,
> ... I am sick and tired of moving around, unless it means a definitive step forward. ... Herefore [!] I cannot risk any more adventures.[15]

And also the move of the Sternbergs to the Rockefeller Institute in New York did not prove to be a great relaxation of their tense living circumstances:

---

[15]Letter of Martin Silberberg (St. Louis) to Leo Loeb (staying at Woodshole) on April-4, 1938; Archives and Rare Books Collection of the Becker Library, Washington University School of Medicine (FC0002, Leo Loeb, Correspondence R-S, Box 5, folder: Silberberg, Martin and Ruth).

Dear Doctor Loeb,

... Nothing has been heard of promotion or raises of salaries, since Dr. [Irving P.] Graef's [1902–1979] departure. I am pretty sure that no changes will take place. It is the policy of the school to exploit everybody and to make use of everybody's plight. The school has the highest percentage of Jewish [!] students, who are glad to pay fees that are about 30% higher than Yale's or Harvard's. On the other hand, the salaries paid to the Faculty are ridiculous. But, what can we do, if the difficulties to obtain a fairly decent position are unsurmountable [!]? The only good aspect is that Dr. [William C.] Von Glahn [1900–1961] lets us have our own ways in research.[16]

This is only one out of many examples that serves to illustrate that the North American context was bursting with all kinds of pragmatic problems, which the newly arriving émigré neuroscientists had to master before they could resume their research and clinical work.

Originality in their scientific work certainly was an important factor to enter major research groups and to gain acceptance in the scientific communities in Canada and the United States. Nevertheless, innovative ideas and the mastering of methods, which were not then accepted in their new host countries, proved to be an ambiguous advantage for the émigrés researchers. An abundant amount of methodological originality, and thus difference in clinical or research style, could easily lead to incommensurable scientific views to those held by the local research community (as in the cases of "holist neurology," the shock therapies in brain psychiatry, or the use of the new psychopharmaceutical drugs, which had yet not been introduced in North America).[17]

Important in this context is that discussions on émigré scientists and physicians had long centered on a preselected group of outstanding individuals, whereas less attention was paid to those more marginal in their field. It is therefore of great importance for further advancement in the historiography of forced migration to draw specific attention to such rather hidden biographies of "normal scientists" and to cases of unsuccessful adaptation in their specific contexts. This will serve the development of a better understanding with regard of the broad transformations and the knowledge transfer in the field of neuroscience. The application of such a perspective will further enable us to also answer such questions as to why it was that the mental health system in Canada and parts of the United States appeared so "underdeveloped" in comparison with the contemporary state of psychiatry and public health in Central Europe. What were the factors that made new research initiatives possible and applicable in the North American contexts? And which factors enabled German-speaking émigrés in particular to overcome everyday problems, research constraints, and cultural differences to contribute to the research traditions of brain psychiatry and clinical neuroscience?

Although this had not been an attractive situation, it was possible to find one individual among the émigrés neuroscientists. An extraordinary pathologist Ruth Silberberg, a Breslau-

---

[16]Letter of Martin Silberberg (NYC) to Leo Loeb (St. Louis) on Dec-2, 1943; Archives and Rare Books Collection of the Becker Library, Washington University School of Medicine (FC0002, Leo Loeb, Correspondence R-S, Box 5, folder: Silberberg, Martin and Ruth).
[17]This made it even harder to find good integration into day-to-day-research work in "normal science" and implies that some narratives will clearly fall into areas of traditional science studies and historical epistemology, as they are current since the works of Thomas S. Kuhn (1962), Georges Canguilhem (1966), Robert K. Merton (1973).

trained developmental brain scientist, who fled with her husband, the neurohistologist Martin Silberberg, first to Halifax and eventually settled in St. Louis, although changing to general pathology during that time. Ruth accepted invitations through the German Pathological Society and individual university institutes to give guest lectures and seminars in Germany during the late 1950s and early 1960s. It was only at the time of Martin's death that she decided to accept an adjunct professorship at the University of Zurich where she frequently taught during the summer break.[18] Ruth Silberberg intriguingly represents an émigré researcher who had an important voice in both medical communities — one that was strongly heard in her own field of pathology as well as in clinical education (cf. Magoun, 2002, p. 151f).

Discussion

As mentioned in the introduction of this article, a more or less unquestioned belief in the historiography of science and medicine at large suggests that the process of forced migration in twentieth-century medicine and natural science can be specifically viewed as a process leading to a "brain gain" of the receiving countries (such as the United States and Canada in North America) (Quirke & Gaudillère, 2008, p. 442). The related view has nearly gone uncontested, namely that it made no difference for a biomedical researcher to substitute Frankfurt am Main for Ottawa, Ontario, Breslau for Halifax, Nova Scotia; or Berlin for Montreal, Quebec, as the respective sites for their research programs and clinical activities. This assumption had some plausibility when compared with the careers of émigré professionals in the arts, in politics, or in the legal sphere (Strauss & Roeder, 1983).

At a second glance, however, the above position of international universality is also not compelling when it is compared with other immigrant groups in the arts and film actors of the Hollywood entertainment industry. In these seemingly unrelated fields, a transfer of knowledge and people could not take place without having to face greater cultural problems (Taylor, 1983, pp. 11–20). The historical analysis of the group of émigré neuroscientists thus presents itself as a most interesting test case for newer approaches in the historiography of science that have interpreted the evolution and aberrations of the biomedical enterprise on grounds of their entanglement with culture. Using historiography as a detailed description of research, laboratory practices, and clinical care approaches allows for a more adequate view of the underlying historical processes, particularly an integration of various communities of neurologists, psychiatrists, and brain investigators into preexisting American research cultures.

In order to come to terms with the cultural differences, which German-speaking émigré neuroscientists experienced when they adapted to North American research and clinical institutions, scientific foundations, and structure of politically influenced forms of research organization, their experiences in the biomedical field at the end of the Weimar Republic and the beginning of the Nazi period in Germany also need to be kept in mind (Roelcke, 2006, pp. 73–87). When considering the transfer of such multifaceted patterns of clinical and basic research, laboratory practices, and interdisciplinary linkages with mental asylums, as well as anthropological research institutions, especially the more hidden biographies and local

---

[18]See in Archives and Rare Books Collection of the Becker Library, Washington University School of Medicine (FC0002, Leo Loeb, Correspondence R-S, Box 5, folder: Silberberg, Martin and Ruth), no page number.

research cultures in the context of the forced migration wave of German-speaking neuroscientists to Canada and the United States, left numerous traces of the setbacks and challenges, which they encountered when they tried to recommence their careers in the North American scientific and clinical milieus. With respect to the case examples discussed in this article, we have seen that the appropriation of new laboratory practices and clinical concepts in the research communities also supported new forms of interdisciplinarity working relations that became so decisive for the neurosciences today. Nevertheless, when looking at the personal experiences, group mentalities, and even the soft skills learned "the hard way," it has likewise become tangible how the research programs of émigré neuroscientists reflected their foregoing experiences in the medical and health care cultures from the late Wilhelminian Empire to the onset of Nazism and Fascism in Central Europe, as well as the problems and setbacks they encountered, when making the very demanding transition to North America and its preexisting research cultures.

References

Anonymous (1993): McGill University, Department of Psychiatry, 50th anniversary. *Journal of Psychiatry and Neuroscience* 18: 141–142.

Argote L (1999): *Organizational Learning: Creating, Retaining, and Transferring Knowledge*. Boston, Kluwer.

Ash MG (2006): Wissens- und Wissenschaftstransfer – Einfuehrende Bemerkungen. *Berichte zur Wissenschaftsgeschichte* 29: 181–189.

Ash M, Soellner A, eds. (1996): *Forced Migration and Scientific Change: Émigré German–speaking Scientists after 1933*. Cambridge, Cambridge University Press.

Bielschowsky M (1933, November 14): Letter to Julius Hallervorden at the KWI for Brain Research in Berlin-Buch. In: Peiffer J, ed., *Hirnforschung in Deutschland 1849 bis 1974. Briefe zur Entwicklung von Psychiatrie und Neurowissenschaften sowie zum Einfluss des politischen Umfeldes auf Wissenschaftler*. Berlin, Springer, p. 496.

Baglole T (2002): Nos disparus—Le Dr Robert Weil, un fondateur de l'APC, est décédé. *Canadian Psychiatric Association Bulletin* 34: 64.

Bullemer T (2003): *"Die hiesigen Juden sind in Cham alteingesessen …": aus der Geschichte der juedischen Gemeinde vom Mittelalter bis zur Gegenwart*. H.Cham, Stadtarchiv.

Canguilhem G (1966): *Le normal et le pathologique*. Paris, Presses Universitaires de France.

Cornwell J (2003): *Hitler's Scientists: Science, War, and the Devil's Pact*. New York, Viking Press.

Dalhousie University (2002, May 15): "In Memoriam Robert Weil." *Dalhousie News*, p. 1.

Danzer G, ed. (2006): *Vom Konkreten zum Abstrakten. Leben und Werk Kurt Goldsteins (1878–1965)*. Frankfurt am Main, Mabuse Verlag.

Davie MR, Koenig S (1949): Adjustment of refugees to American life. *Annals of the American Academy of Political and Social Science* 262: 159–165.

Deichmann U (1996): *Biologists under Hitler*. Cambridge, MA, Harvard University Press.

Dowbiggin IR (2003): *Keeping America Sane: Psychiatry and Eugenics in North America and Canada, 1880–1940*. New York, Cornell University Press.

Erickson M (2005): *Science, Culture and Society: Understanding Science in the Twenty-First Century*. Cambridge, England, Cambridge University Press.

Feindel W (1984): The contributions of Wilder Penfield and the Montreal Neurological Institute to Canadian neurosciences. In: Roland CC, ed., *Health, Disease and Medicine*. Toronto, Hannah Institute for the History of Medicine, pp. 347–358.

Feindel W (1991): The Montreal Neurological Institute. *Journal of Neurosurgery* 75: 821–822.

Fischer K (1996): Identification of emigration-induced scientific change. In: Ash M, Soellner A, eds., *Forced Migration and Scientific Change. Émigré German-Speaking Scientists and Scholars after 1933*. Cambridge, Cambridge University Press, 1996, pp. 23–47.

Galison P, Graubard SR, Mendelsohn E, eds. (2001): *Science in Culture*. New Brunswick, NJ, London, Harvard University Press.

Goldblatt D (1992): Star: Karl Stern (1906–1975). *Seminars in Neurology* 12: 279–282.

Grob GN (1983): *Mental Illness and American Society, 1875–1940*. Princeton, NJ, Princeton University Press.

Grossmann A (1993): German women doctors from Berlin to New York: Maternity and modernity in Weimar and in exile. *Feminist Studies* 19: 65–88.

Hammerstein N (2000): *Die Deutsche Forschungsgemeinschaft in der Zeit der Weimarer Republik und im Dritten Reich; Wissenschaftspolitik in Republik und Diktatur*. Munich, C. H. Beck.

Harrington A (1991): *Reenchanted Science: Holism in German Culture from Wilhelm II to Hitler*. Princeton, NJ, Princeton University Press, 2nd edition.

Hincks CM (1947): Canadian psychiatry. *Canadian Medical Association Journal* 57: 161–165.

Hogan D (2007): History of geriatrics in Canada. *Canadian Bulletin of Medical History* 24: 131–150.

Holdorff B (2016): Emigrated neuroscientists from Berlin to North America. *Journal of the History of the Neurosciences* 25: 227–252.

Israel G (2004): Science and the Jewish question in the twentieth century: The case of Italy and what it shows. *Aleph. Historical Studies in Science and Judaism* 2: 191–261.

Jankrift KP, Steger F, eds. (2004), *Gesundheit – Krankheit. Kulturtransfer medizinischen Wissens von der Spaetantike bis in die Fruehe Neuzeit*. Koeln, Boehlau.

Juette R (1990): *Die Emigration der deutschsprachigen "Wissenschaft des Judentums". Die Auswanderung juedischer Historiker nach Palaestina 1933–1945*. Stuttgart, Franz Steiner.

Kreft G (1997): Zwischen Goldstein und Kleist: Zum Verhaeltnis von Neurologie und Psychiatrie in Frankfurt am Main der 1920er Jahre. *Schriftenreihe der Deutschen Gesellschaft fuer Geschichte der Nervenheilkunde* 3: 131–144.

Kuhn TS (1962): *The Structure of Scientific Revolutions*. Chicago, Chicago University Press.

Kuhn TS (1977): *The Essential Tension: Selected Studies in Scientific Tradition and Change*. Chicago, University of Chicago Press.

Laier M (1994): Kurt Goldstein: Zur Erinnerung an einen vergessenen Neurologen. In: Wilmans, ed., *Medizin in Frankfurt am Main. Ein Symposium zum 65. Geburtstag von Gert Preiser*. Hildesheim, Olms-Weidmann, pp. 176–186.

Lehmann H (1983): Zur Casuistik des Inducirten Irreseins (Folie à deux). *Archiv fuer Psychiatrie und Neurologie* 1: 145–154.

Lunbeck E (1995): *The Psychiatric Persuasion: Knowledge, Gender, and Power in Modern America*. Princeton, Princeton University Press.

Magoun HW (2002): *American Neuroscience in the Twentieth Century: Confluence of the Neural, Behavioral, and Communicative Streams*, edited and annotated by Louise H. Marshall. Lisse, A. A. Balkema Publishers.

Medawar J, Pyke D (2001): *Hitler's Gift: The True Story of the Scientists Expelled by the Nazi Regime*. New York, Arkade Publishing.

Medical Research Council (MRC) (2000): *Celebrating the Medical Research Council of Canada – A Voyage in Time, 1960–2000*. Ottawa, Medical Research Council of Canada.

Merton RK (1973): *The Sociology of Science*. Chicago, Chicago University Press.

Meyer JB (2001): Network approach versus brain drain: Lessons from the diaspora. *International Migration* 39: 91–110.

Pearle KM (1984): Aerzteemigration nach 1933 in die USA: Der Fall New York. *Medizinhistorisches Journal* 19: 112–137.

Peiffer J (1998a): Die Vertreibung deutscher Neuropathologen 1933–1939. *Der Nervenarzt* 69: 99–109.

Peiffer J (1998b): Zur Neurologie im "Dritten Reich" und ihren Nachwirkungen. *Der Nervenarzt* 69: 728–733.

Peiffer J (1998c): Neuropathology in the Third Reich. *Epidemiologia e prevenzione* 22: 184–190.

Peiffer J (2004): *Hirnforschung in Deutschland 1849 bis 1974. Briefe zur Entwicklung von Psychiatrie und Neurowissenschaften sowie zum Einfluss des politischen Umfeldes auf Wissenschaftler*. Berlin, Springer.

Quirke V, Gaudillère JP (2008): The era of biomedicine: Science, medicine, and public health in Britain and France after the Second World War. *Medical History* 52: 441–452.

Rheinberger HJ (2005): Reassessing the historical epistemology of Georges Canguilhem. In: Gutting G, ed., *Continental Philosophy of Science*. Maldan, MA, Blackwell Publishing, pp. 187–197.

Roelcke V (2006): Funding the scientific foundations of race policies: Ernst Ruedin and the impact of career resources on psychiatric genetics, ca. 1910–1945. In: Eckart WU, ed., *Man, Medicine, and the State: The Human Body as an Object of Government Sponsored Medical Research in the 20th Century*. Stuttgart, Franz Steiner, pp. 73–87.

Rosen G (1944): *The Specialization of Medicine with Particular Reference to Ophthalmology*. New York, Froben Press.

Sachs L (1998): Advice from the Midwest. In: Anderson MM, ed., *Hitler's Exiles. Personal Stories of the Fight from Nazi Germany to America*. New York, The New Press, pp. 229–232.

Schmidgen H, Geimer P, Dierig S, eds. (2004): *Kultur im Experiment*. Berlin, Cadmos.

Seidelman W (2000): The legacy of academic medicine and human exploitation in the Third Reich. *Perspectives in Biology and Medicine* 43: 325–334.

Soellner A (1996): *Deutsche Politikwissenschaftler in der Emigration. Ihre Akkulturation und Wirkungsgeschichte, samt einer Bibliographie*. Opladen, Westdeutscher Verlag.

Sourkes TL, Pinard G, eds. (1995): *Building on a Proud Past: 50 Years of Psychiatry at McGill*. Montreal, McGill University, Douglas Hospital.

Stahnisch FW (2008): Ludwig Edinger (1855–1918) – Pioneer in Neurology. *Journal of Neurology* 255: 147–148.

Stahnisch FW (2010): German–speaking émigré–neuroscientists in North America after 1933: Critical reflections on emigration–induced scientific change. *Oesterreichische Zeitschrift fuer Geschichtswissenschaften* (Vienna) 21: 36–68.

Stahnisch FW, Pow S (2014): Walther Riese (1890–1976) – Pioneer in Neurology. *Journal of Neurology* 261: 2466–2468.

Stahnisch FW, Pow S (2015): Karl Stern (1906–1975) – Pioneer of Neurology. *Journal of Neurology* 262: 245–247.

Stern K (1951): *The Pillar of Fire*. New York, Harcourt, Brace, and Company.

Stern K (1939): Severe dementia associated with bilateral symmetrical degeneration of the thalamus. *Brain* 62: 157–167.

Stip E (2015): Who pioneered the use of antipsychotoics in North America? *Canadian Journal of Psychiatry* 60: S5–S13.

Stortz P (2003): "Rescue our family from a living death": Refugee professors and the Canadian Society for the Protection of Science and Learning at the University of Toronto, 1935–1946. *Journal of the Canadian Historical Association* 14: 231–261.

Strauss HA, Roeder W, eds. (1983): *International Biographical Dictionary of Central European Emigrés 1933–1945*. The Arts, Sciences, and Literature. 2 Volumes. Munich, K. G. Saur.

Taylor JR (1983): *Strangers in Paradise: The Hollywood Émigrés 1933–1950*. New York, Holt Rinehart and Winston.

Weber MM (2000): Psychiatric research and science policy in Germany: The history of the Deutsche Forschungsanstalt fuer Psychiatrie (German Institute for Psychiatric Research) in Munich from 1917 to 1945. *History of Psychiatry* 11: 235–258.

Weil RJ (1960): Mental health and disasters. In: Baker GW, Rohrer JH, eds., *Symposium in Human Problems in the Utilization of Fallout Shelters*. Washington, DC, Disaster Research Group.

Weil RJ, Demay M (1947): Thiamine chloride intrathecally. *Canadian Medical Association Journal* 56: 545–456.

Weindling PJ (1989): *Health, Race and German Politics between National Unification and Nazism, 1870–1945*. Cambridge, Cambridge University Press.

Zeidman LA (2014): Adolf Wallenberg: Giant in neurology and refugee from Nazi Europe. *Journal of the History of the Neurosciences* 23: 31–44.

Zimmerman D (2006): The Society for the Protection of Science and Learning and the Politization of British Science in the 1930s. *Minerva* 44: 25–45.

A variation on forced migration: Wilhelm Peters (Prussia via Britain to Turkey) and Muzafer Sherif (Turkey to the United States)

Gül A. Russell

ABSTRACT

In 1933 the Turkish Republic formally offered university positions to 30 German-speaking academics who were dismissed with the coming to power of the National Socialist Government. That initial number went up to 56 with the inclusion of the technical assistants. By 1948 the estimated total had increased to 199. Given renewable five-year contracts with salaries substantially higher than their Turkish counterparts, the foreign émigrés were to implement the westernization program of higher education. The ten year-old secular Turkish Republic's extensive social reforms had encompassed the adoption of the Latin alphabet, and equal rights for women, removing gender bias in hiring. Such a high concentration of émigré academics in one institution, "the highest anywhere in the world," provides a unique opportunity to study a subject which has been neglected. In this article two cases in psychology will be examined: Wilhelm Peters (1880–1963), who came, via Britain, to Istanbul in 1936 from the University of Jena in Germany, and Muzafer Sherif (1906–1988) who went to the United States from Ankara University in 1945. The purpose of the comparative analysis is to identify the features that are specific to the German experience, and those that are shared and underlie translocation in science within the multifaceted complexity of the process of forced migration.

Psychology has a long past but a short history.
(Hermann Ebbinghaus, 1908, p. 2)

Introduction

It is hardly known that in 1933, following the dismissal of prominent academics from their posts with the coming to power of the National Socialist Party, Istanbul University acquired the highest number of German speaking academics at a single institution anywhere in the world (Epstein, 1998). On this basis alone (see Fig. 1), case of the Turkish Republic has a significant place in the history of the forced migration of neurologists, psychiatrists, and neuropathologists during the time of Nazism and Fascism in Europe, with special features that are both unique and relate to others. It is unique because when individual scientists and physicians who had been forced to leave their positions under the Nazis in 1933 were facing

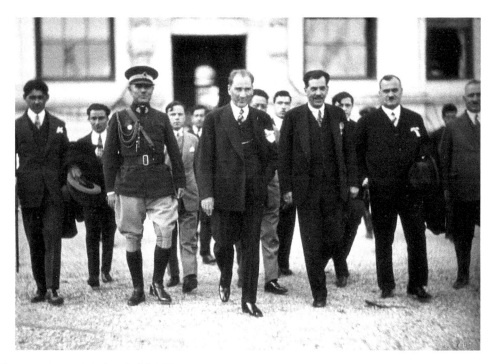

Figure 1. Atatuerk in Istanbul (1932).

insurmountable difficulties in trying to get into other countries, the Turkish Republic had officially offered highly paid, salaried positions with three- to five-year contracts to initially 30 distinguished academics (largely Jewish), with numbers steadily increasing until 1945. In fact, out of the estimated 650 scientists, clinicians, and neurological scholars, who left Germany between 1933–1945, 190 went to Turkey. This is 29% of the total (Bentwich, 1953). They were allowed to bring their families and possessions, along with their technicians, assistants, and equipment. They survived the war, and subsequently moved to the United States with some choosing to remain, and others even returning to Germany. Yet, this phenomenon seems to have received little attention in the English-speaking scholarship of the subject prior to the twenty-first century, and then with some exceptions, only sporadically, without sufficient research or rigorous analysis. This in itself raises challenging questions about the nature of historiographical scholarship. This article for the *Journal of the History of the Neurosciences* special issue provides an opportunity to rectify the current gap in the literature. There is a great wealth of unpublished original documents, particularly from the rich government and university archives, in addition to personal correspondence and published diaries. For example, the holdings of the two key institutions, the Istanbul and Ankara University Medical Schools, are crucial concerning émigré academics for the period 1933–1970.[1]

Despite the cultural divide and level of scientific knowledge at the time, the experiences of the émigrés in Turkey show remarkable similarities across the board with North America. The comparative exploration of the common threads has profound implications for our under-standing of the broader fundamental questions embodied in the "brain drain" (Medawar &

---

[1]One of the key scholars who has extensively publicized the subject in numerous books and articles is Arnold Riesman.

Pyke, 2001, p. 7), going beyond the upheaval caused by the Nazis: For example, what happens to such scientists themselves, as well as to their "science" in new environments (whether receptive or hostile); how do they affect their new milieus; what are the losses and gains? Such questions will be taken up by analyzing the experiences of two psychologists: Wilhelm Peters (1880–1963), who came, via Britain, to Istanbul in 1936 after being dismissed from the University of Jena in Prussia. To extend the subject beyond the specific focus on forced migration due to Nazi Germany, a comparable second case will be examined with Muzafer Sherif (1906–1988) who was forced to leave Ankara University and went to the United States in 1945. In revealing the levels of complexity in what is usually posed in terms merely of "transmission and reception of knowledge," the research would be a significant enduring contribution.[2]

Wilhelm Peters in Britain: Desperate years

Not a country but a staging post.
(Walther Gropius, quoted in McKibbin, 1998, p. 256)

Wilhelm Peters (1880–1963)[3] was in the first wave of leading psychologists to be relieved of their university positions under the "Law for the Re-establishment for a Professional Civil Service" (1933, April 7). He had held the first chair of experimental psychology at the University of Jena in Germany and two years later the directorship of the Institute of Psychology at its founding in 1925 (Holzapfel, 2001).

   Peters was able to move first to Britain, then in 1937 to Turkey through the efforts of Phillip Schwartz (1894–1977; see Fig. 2), the former professor of neuropathology at Frankfurt am Main and the founder of the *Notgemeinschaft Deutscher Wissenschaftler* [Emergency Assistance Association (ACC) for German Scientists] in Zurich in March 1933. He was also working together with the Academic Assistance Council in Britain (Schwartz, 1995; Kreft, 2011). Wilhelm Peters (Fig. 3) together with David Katz (1884–1953) were the two full

---

[2]My own interest in the subject had long been gestating since my encounter, as a graduate student in Bloomington, Indiana, with Felix Michael Haurowitz (1896–1987), the distinguished biochemist and Fellow of the American Academy of Science, who had survived the war years at the University of Istanbul in Turkey and continued his close academic and personal ties with the country. In a more recent past, at a commemorative meeting held at Istanbul Medical School, I became aware of the extensive role of the "German-Physicians in Turkey (1933–48)" (see also Reisman, 2008). A further stimulus was the personal account of a descendent, a psychiatrist in Geneva, Switzerland, the initial starting point of the exiled émigrés who took up academic posts at the University of Istanbul on the official invitation of the Turkish Republic. The discovery of a letter by Albert Einstein, addressed to the Turkish Prime Minister in 1933, unfolded another layer (Reisman, 2006). Subsequently, an invited lectureship, sponsored by Public Partnership & Outreach, Office of the Provost, at Texas A&M University in 2014, provided an additional opportunity to present my findings and analysis within the context of Turkey's Higher Education Reforms, involving specifically the biomedical and brain sciences. Two specific cases are presented here in this article.

[3]The following discussion is based on the unpublished correspondence in the Bodleian Library Archives between Wilhelm Peters, the British Academic Assistance Council (ACC), and the British Home Office during a period from October 26, 1934 to October 3, 1936. Despite gaps, there is sufficient detail to gain a clear picture of Peters' experience in Britain. This is not an exhaustive research on Peters or his stay in Britain, but highlights what is relevant to the overall theme of this special issue. (Henceforth, it will be cited as AAC-W. Peters, 1934–1936).

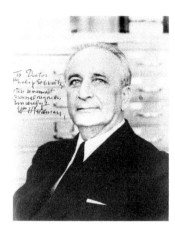

Figure 2. Phillip Schwartz.

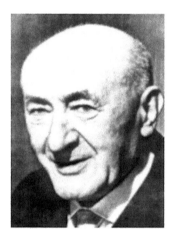

Figure 3. Wilhelm Peters.

professors among the relatively few but important émigré psychologists to go to Britain. After three years, however, both had to leave due to a lack of continued financial support and the prospect of a permanent job, which Britain was not in any position to offer for a number of complex reasons (Geuter, 1992; Ash & Soellner, 1996).

Peters' experience in Britain highlights those of the individually placed émigré academics, the criteria of their selection, and provides a basis of comparison with his subsequent stay at Istanbul University in Turkey that lasted 16 years (from 1937 to 1952) until his return to Germany as an Emeritus Professor at the University of Wuerzburg.

The role of the Maudsley Hospital

In Britain, Peters' position was temporary and not commensurate with his professional seniority. The financial support by various organizations, such as the British Academic Assistance Council, and the Home Office permit to stay served only as stopgap measures until finding a permanent position in Britain or elsewhere. As the only opportunities and support for the émigrés in Britain were more in clinical and applied fields (U. H. Peters,

1996), particularly in psychology (Ash, 1991).[4] Peters had to undertake observational research at child clinics and various mental asylums without a fixed position, moving from one institution to another. From the reference in his correspondence, he appears to have been sponsored by Frederick Lucien Golla (1877–1968),[5] neurophysiologist, and director of the Central Pathology Laboratory at the Maudsley Hospital in London, Chair of the Medical Research Council's Mental Disorder Committee, and the honorary director of the Maudsley Hospital Medical School since 1923 (Jones, Rahman, & Woolven, 2007).

Maudsley was receptive to German émigrés for self-serving reasons. With the ambitious aim of raising the status of academic psychiatry and neurology within the United Kingdom, the Maudsley Hospital was designed to address the effective treatment of major mental illness, which was originally inspired by a visit in 1904 to Emil Kraepelin's (1856–1926) institute of psychiatry in Munich. It was also to provide facilities for postgraduate training (Jones, Rahman, & Woolven 2007). At the time, the major problem for the Maudsley Hospital was how to get funding as a research center for the scientific and experimental study of neurosis and mental illness without a track record of published research and internationally recognized clinicians, with Golla as the only possible exception. Golla also believed that the means to understand severe psychological disorders was through the study of brain physiology. The émigré medical scientists from Germany offered an opportunity to enhance the institute's needed international research visibility to secure funds from the Rockefeller Foundation (Jones & Rahman, 2009).

Thus, Peters conducted clinical observational research at the Maudsley Hospital, and at its associated Child Guidance Clinic, where changes were being introduced in theory, practice, and methods of treatment were being introduced. For example, the concept of "behavior disorder" was replacing traditional diagnoses of delinquent children.[6] Such work was only partly related to Peters' interest in individual differences in child and adolescent development. He had some clinical training in psychiatry under Kraepelin in Munich, but that was more than two decades earlier in 1906 and 1907 (Holzapfel, 2001). Since the 1920s, however, Peters had been among the few psychologists who were not only conducting experiments, using quantitative and statistical methods, but who had directed their scientific interest to the service of school reform, and social projects (Ash, 2013). This background may also account for the nature of Peters' employment in Britain.

---

[4]In fact, some of those who were able to remain seem to have shifted their careers accordingly to clinical areas (Carlebach, et al., 1991; U. H. Peters, 1996).

[5]Frederick Golla had a distinguished record. He was elected president of the neurology and psychiatry section of the Royal Society of Medicine, president of the Electroencephalographic Society, and of the Society for the Study of Addiction. He was also a member of the Royal Medico-Psychological Association. In 1937, he was appointed professor of mental pathology at the University of London, as well as conducting important clinical studies (histological, chemical, and electro-physiological) at Maida Vale Hospital. Thus, Golla was influential having both academic status and financial security (see Jones, Rahman, & Woolven, 2007).

[6]In the "General Articles and News Section" of May 30, 1936, the *British Medical Journal* has the following on the East London Child Guidance Clinic: "This clinic held a demonstration of work and methods of treatment with diagrams, and statistics at the Jews' Free School on May 18th on its value to the child patients and to the community at large, (Lecture), with delinquent children, importance of understanding the relation of mind/body, and behavior and adaptation to their surroundings to enhance a new understanding of the child and mental problems by society" (Anonymous, 1936, p. 1123).

University College links to the University of Wuerzburg

It is mentioned that Peters was also engaged in research in 1934 at the University College London's Psychological Laboratory, as well as giving ad hoc lectures (Kravetz, 1993). There is, however, no further information.[7] Historically the University College London faculty also had links through psychology with the Universities of Leipzig and Wuerzburg, where Peters was a *"Privatdozent"* from 1910 to 1919 and a full professor (*Ordentlicher Professor*) from 1919 to 1923 in the psychology departments before moving to Jena where he stayed until his dismissal in 1933.

John Carl Fluegel (1884–1955), who was at the time directing the psychological laboratories at University College London, had studied experimental psychology at the University of Wuerzburg, using the new statistical methods introduced by Charles Edward Spearman (1863–1945). He was a strong promoter of the study of psychology and its acceptance as a science (Jensen, 1994). Charles Edward Spearman too had studied experimental psychology and received his PhD under Wilhelm Wundt (1832–1920) at Leipzig in 1906, and he worked with the structural psychologist Oswald Kuelpe (1862–1915) at the University of Würzburg. Peters, as a pioneer of IQ (Intelligence Quotient) testing, would have been familiar with Spearman's work that introduced the statistical method of two-factor analysis, providing the theoretical justification for intelligence testing (Weiss, 1980). Although Spearman had retired in 1931, through his influence and the popularization of Cyril Burt (1883–1971) (see Fig. 4) University College London had become the center of psychological studies in Britain, associated with systematic testing and statistical methods, also rooted in Francis Galton (1822–1911) and Karl Pearson (1857–1936) in the context of eugenics. Even with such connections what had been secured for Peters was no more than a tenuous affiliation.

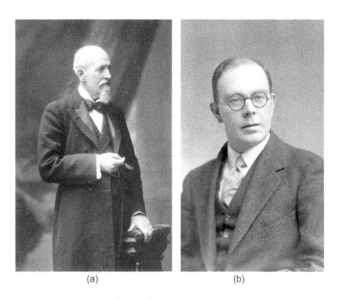

(a)   (b)

Figure 4. (a) Charles Edward Spearman (1863–1945). (b) Cyril Burt (1883–1971).

---

[7]A statement in Peters' correspondence that the "Secretary of State does not raise any objection to Dr. W. Peters engaging in research work at UCL" suggests an application for rather than an on-going work. See AAC File-W. Peters (1934 November 8).

Furthermore, Peters was not an unfamiliar figure as a member of the British Psychological Association, and at least through the *British Medical Journal* (Weiss, 1980). At the same time, one has to bear in mind that with the paucity of academic posts, applications for lectureships were discouraged by the Academic Assistance Council to avoid unfair competition for the junior faculty (Carlebach, 1991; McKibbin, 1998).

Clinical peregrinations

The observational research took Peters to numerous mental asylums in and around London (Southgate London, Cayne/Cane Hill, Coulsdon, Camstock, and Epsom, etc.), living in hotels near the institutions where he worked. Thus, he had no fixed address as it kept changing accordingly.[8] Correspondence suggests that the observational work was part of a project under Golla, who was critical of the traditional methods of treatment used at the Maudsley Hospital.[9]

In addition to the intermittent nature of the work, Peters was also constantly struggling to have his stay extended by the Home Office at intervals of six months to a year, for which he needed to provide both a justification of his clinical research and evidence of funding to be able to support him. On one occasion, he had to take a leave of absence outside Britain ("on vacation") as advised and then return to get an approval of stay. He was plagued by constant fear of losing his passport, not having it renewed, or taken by the German authorities.[10]

The criteria for extension of stay are clearly stated in the Home Office response to the British Academic Assistance Council: as long as Peters "does not take employment paid or unpaid other than his research work at the Maudsley hospital and at such centers where it may be necessary for him to undertake clinical observational work."[11] Peter's case appears to exemplify the restrictions under which the émigré academics were employed in Britain, as well as the emphasis on applied clinical work (U. H. Peters, 1996). In the spring of 1936, Peters was still uncertain as to where he would go in the coming months ("to another mental asylum" or "back to the Maudsley"). He was reduced to proving support by personal funds, which came from friends in Czechoslovakia and was organized through a daily quota to his bank. Golla's attempts to get Peters' Rockefeller funding had failed, which also meant the failure of the original rationale for his sponsorship by the Maudsley Hospital. Ongoing funding by the British Academic Assistance Council was out of the question. His permit was extended only until October 1936.

Peter's experiences in Britain are characterized by desperate financial difficulties, constant insecurity due to the temporary nature of the support, and visa extension as a stopgap measure until finding a permanent position in Britain or elsewhere when neither one was forthcoming. This was also true for a figure like David Katz (1884–1953), who had the

---

[8]AAC File:W. Peters (October 26, 1934–October 29, 1935).
[9]For the Maudsleys' involvement with eugenics and the related psychiatric treatments, see Mazumdar (2005).
[10]AAC File:W. Peters (October 26, 1934–October 29, 1935).
[11]AAC File:W. Peters (September 23, 1936).

positive testimonials of leading psychologists and educators, such as Cyril Burt (1883–1971) of the University College London, to evaluate the practical value of his work and even the positive assets of his personality (Geuter, 1992; Ash & Soellner, 1996). Curiously, Burt did not mention Peters.[12]

The final recommendation of the British Academic Assistance Council and the Home Office was for Peters to return to Germany, clearly based also on the consideration of his advanced age, where he was entitled to a retirement pension, and wait there.[13] With no future prospects or further funding, Peter's situation had become bleak.

The Turkish Republic: Another chance?

An invitation cabled from the Turkish Republic on September 14, 1936, was most timely for a position at Istanbul University (Ash & Soellner, 1996). The recruitment of academics by the Turkish government was still continuing after their offer in 1933 of 30 initial contractual positions. No recommendations had been made in 1933 (Bentwich, 1936). In 1936, the chair of experimental psychology was still vacant.[14] It was an offer which Peters could not refuse. In contrast to the uncertainty of his British situation, he now had a five-year contract at Istanbul University (see Fig. 5) effective from January 15, 1937, to January 1, 1942, which was periodically renewed until 1952.

Peters was the third choice after the experimental psychologist Adhémar Gelb (1887–1936) of Halle University, who died, and the psychologist and educator David Katz of Rostock, who took up the alternative offer from Stockholm, Sweden (Brock, 1992). Peters was much more suited for the needs of the discipline at Istanbul University and the obligations as outlined in his contract by the Turkish Government (Doelen, 2010) in terms of his qualifications. He had been a professor of experimental psychology since 1923 and headed the psychological laboratory since its foundation in 1925 at Jena University. His work was in the field of educational and developmental psychology (especially the nature-nurture problem) and intelligence testing that he pioneered in Germany (Holzapfel, 2005). In addition, he had been in the center of the institutionalization of psychology as a professional discipline during the Weimar Period to which he had made a significant contribution at Jena. He also came from a university system centralized by the state, as exemplified by his appointment to the first chair of psychology at Jena against the wishes of the philosophy faculty (Eckardt, 2003).

---

[12]Burt's correspondence at University College archives may reveal whether or not he had any role in the selection of Peters' employment. The opening of the London Child Guidance Clinic in Islington in 1927 was largely due to the influence of Burt's 1925 publication, *The Young Delinquent*. He had carried out his child guidance work as Professor of Educational Psychology in 1924 at the London Day Training College, a teacher-training college, associated with the University of London (Aldrich, 2002). Peter was familiar with Burt's work.

[13]AAC File: W. Peters (September 23, 1936).

[14]The number of psychologists and psychiatrists who came to Turkey was very small in comparison with medicine and other disciplines. Peters is the only psychologist listed (Widman, 1973) out of 120 émigré psychologists, with the majority (80) going to the USA (Ash & Soellner, 1996). There were, however, psychiatrists, such as Edith Weigert (1894–1982) in Ankara who subsequently flourished in the USA. See Holmes (2010).

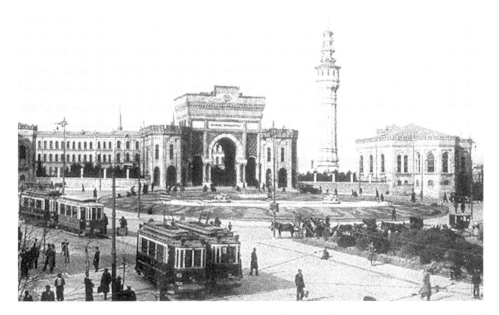

Figure 5. Istanbul University (1930s): The former Daruelfuenun, the Ottoman Institution of higher education.

Furthermore, the place of professional psychology, outside the United States, was not clearly determined, hovering between the natural sciences and the humanities in the period between the two world wars in Germany as well as Britain. Peters' chair was located in the Faculty of Mathematics and Natural Sciences (Ash, 2015). Earlier, for example, Peters' doctoral dissertation on *Die Farbenwahrnehmung der Netzhautperipherie* (Color Perception on the Periphery of the Retina), completed in 1904 under Wundt (1832–1920) and Wiener in Leipzig, and his habilitation in 1910 at the University of Wuerzburg were both from institutes of psychology but within the Faculty of Philosophy (W. Peters, 1904).

Istanbul University: Continuity from Jena — Unbroken?

Psychology has a long past, yet its real history is short.
(Ebbinghaus, 1908, p. 3)

At Istanbul University, Peters faced an analogous situation where his chair in experimental psychology was in the Department of Philosophy (Doelen, 2010). With his prior experience, Peters could address institutional development of psychology as an independent academic discipline. Thus, considering that "few émigré Central European Jewish psychologists [who] found academic or professional positions from which they could have engaged in transfers of their scientific knowledge or other skills" (Carlebach, 1991, p. 107), the appointment seemed a unique match. What Peters could not, however, have envisaged the extent of the formidable difficulties he would encounter due to the gap between his expectations on the basis of his own background, and the cultural operational reality in his new environment.[15]

The progress report on the "Institute of Pedagogy 1937–43," which he prepared as Director of the Pedagogical and Psychological Institute six years after his appointment. He first summarizes what was initially expected of him. These were (a) to establish the institute (which had been planned in 1936 prior to his arrival), (b) to train and prepare future instructors/school teachers; and (c) to teach philosophy students experimental psychology, "a subject which [as he put it] at present appears to occupy the whole area of modern psychology" (Peters, 1952a, pp. 5–6). What he found in psychology was complex but lacking in research. The continental developments in psychology had in part been imported in the first two decades of the twentieth century through faculty who had been sent abroad. They were idiosyncratically representing French and German influences according to their training at the J. J Rousseau Institute in Switzerland and the University of Frankfurt am Main.[16]

Experimental psychology had been introduced prior to World War One as a consequence of the Wilhelmian policy (1897–1914) of the German government to promote German cultural and philological influences in order to strengthen its alliance with Turkey. Ostensibly to help reform the existing Ottoman institution, the *Daruelfuenun*, with the underlying intention to minimize the traditional French influence, they had sent the 20 academics in various disciplines, from 1913 to 1915. Among them, Georg Anschuetz (1886–1953) from the Department of Philosophy at the University of Hamburg, and a former assistant to Ernst Meumann (1862–1915), was appointed as professor of pedagogy and experimental psychology. He was trained at Leipzig, Munich, Wuerzburg, and Berlin, including a year at Alfred Binet's (1857–1911) laboratory in Paris. Yet, Anschuetz does not seem to have left much of a legacy for his three-year stay. The Research Institute for Experimental Psychology that he started, with an assistant and some imported equipment, was closed after his departure at the outbreak of the First World War (Widmann, 1973; Batur 2002; 2005). Despite his efforts, the failure of Anschuetz to establish experimental

---

[15]Peters does not describe the actual obligations in his contract. In the first three years, he could conduct his lectures in a foreign language, then switch to Turkish and write a textbook on psychology. He was also required to educate schoolteachers, give additional public lectures and help develop cultural institutions in areas related to psychology and pedagogy. His salary was set, although not comparable to that of his colleagues in medicine and the sciences. Upon his complaint of its inadequacy, it was rectified based on his position as "Institute Director." He was also provided with health insurance (W. Peters, 1949; Doelen, 2007; 2010). With the salary raise, he was able to bring his family: his wife, his daughter, and his son, Georg, who completed his medical degree at Istanbul Medical School under the tutelage of the German-speaking medical faculty in 1943, and worked in Turkey until 1947 (Batur, 2002).

[16]Prior to Wilhelm Peters, Mustafa Şekip Tunç (1866–1958), educated at the J. J. Rousseau Institute in Switzerland, is regarded as the founder of psychology at Istanbul University. In 1919, he had published a translation of Hermann Ebbinghaus' (1850–1909) *"Psychologie."* His main interest was in Henri Bergson (1859–1941) and Sigmund Freud (1856–1939), not in experimental psychology (Toğrol, 1987). Peters (1944) subsequently appraised him, however, of introducing psychological terminology.

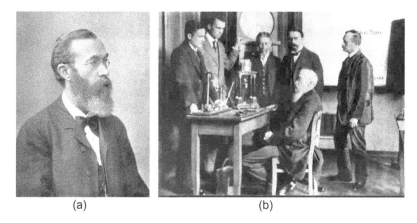

(a)   (b)

Figure 6. (a) Wilhelm Wundt (1832–1920). (b) Wilhelm Wundt with his research group.

psychology exemplifies the complexity of transplanting a discipline without the necessary conditions to establish roots (McKinney, 1960).[17]

For Wilhelm Peters, the contrast between his own former milieu — even after the British interlude, as described above — must have been painfully obvious, creating at times insurmountable difficulties in his relationship with the Turkish faculty, administration, staff, and the central authority of the state. Peters was a product of the Weimar Period that is described as the "crucible of intellectual innovation," an astonishing cultural and intellectual ferment of interwar Germany between 1919 and 1933 (Ash, 2015, p. 2). He was trained and worked at major German institutions—Frankfurt am Main, Leipzig, Wuerzburg, and finally at Jena (W. Peters, 1904). He was mentored by, and colleague of, the leading experimental, gestalt, and developmental psychologists in Germany (see Figs. 6–8), such as Wilhelm Wundt (1832–1920), Max Wertheimer (1880–1943), Carl Marbe (1869–1953), David Katz (1880–1953), Kurt Lewin (1890–1947), Adhémar Gelb (1887–1936), Kurt Koffka (1886–1943), and Wilhelm Koehler (1887–1967). Their exodus (the "brain drain") has, in fact, been viewed as bringing about a total decline of psychology, justified though not entirely true, under the Nazis (Mandler & Mandler, 1969; Geuter 1992).

In his new environment the culture was unfamiliar, the language outside Peters' proficiency (Greek, Latin, French, Italian, English), and the university milieu, lacking in a tradition of scientific research. On the surface such a milieu would not have been intellectually challenging for him. The language barrier, which is usually mentioned as a major problem for émigré academics and scientists (Widmann, 1973), was somewhat minimized, but not entirely removed. Peters could communicate in French, English, as well as in German with his assistants and some of the faculty who were trained abroad. They translated his articles and lectures, and some of the needed key texts for teaching and research training purposes. For not learning Turkish, as dictated by the terms of his contract, he was subsequently criticized by some of the faculty with the pressure of increasing nationalism. In Germany, Peters had been involved in the emerging institutionalization of psychology as "part of a school reform movement," where the

---

[17]Courses in developmental and educational psychology, testing and measurement were already being offered at the Teacher Training Institute in Ankara in 1923 (W. Peters, 1952a).

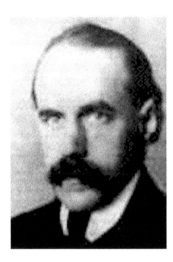

Figure 7. Max Wertheimer (1880–1943).

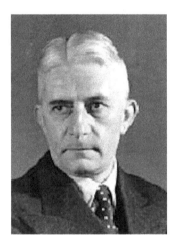

Figure 8. Wilhelm Koehler (1887–1967).

university system was also state organized (Geuter, 1992, p. 4).[18] Interestingly, the policy of the Turkish Ministry of education was analogous to that of the Prussian State in its emphasis on the need to train teachers. Peters was thus to use psychology as an "educational science" at Istanbul University. Peters promoted the need to focus on training teachers, not simply teach psychology to philosophy students alone (W. Peters, 1952b).

His pessimism was hardly disguised in describing the history of the Institute of Pedagogy, despite his efforts and considerable achievements (1937–1943) over 6 years. Although more than 60 studies were conducted in 16 areas of research, they were not all up to publishable level (W. Peters, 1943). The difficulties he faced in training students arose from the absence of a proper foundation in a scientific tradition and of indigenous role models. He states that:

---

[18]In supporting psychology at institutions of teacher colleges psychologists viewed it as a chance to get professorships as well as teacher training (Geuter, 1992).

One who has not learned how to conduct scientific experiments, can never do scientific research. … To learn the technique of writing scientific research is difficult when there are no models in one's own language no matter how many foreign ones are available. (W. Peters, 1943, p. 8)

What Peters stated, a decade after the report on higher education in Turkey by Dr. Albert Malche (1876–1856) from Sweden in 1932, still confirmed its findings of passive rote learning, the lack of scientific research, and faculty publications (Peters, 1940). His attempts to rectify the situation for the next generation of students were accomplished through the establishment of a laboratory with equipment imported from abroad, the establishment of a library of important books, some of which were translated into Turkish by his assistants, and by subscribing to leading international psychology journals, and expanding the curriculum (Batur, 2002; Toğrol, 1983).

The journal that Peters established and edited in Istanbul, entitled *Studies in Psychology and Pedagogy (from the Institute of Pedagogy)*, exemplifies how he used his prior academic and administrative experiences before emigrating to Turkey. The first issue, which appeared in 1940, contains brief reports similar to his journal at the University of Wuerzburg, the *Zentralblatt fuer Psychologie und psychologische Paedagogik* [Archive of Psychology and Psychological Pedagogy], contained no original investigations but only abstracts and reviews. Its aim was to cover the whole field, pure as well as applied, with special attention to educational psychology, and to provide a comprehensive report on recent publications in any part of the psychological field. The rationale of the German model was thus fundamentally different. The format and style of such a journal seemed appropriate to booster and advance the state of research at the Istanbul Institute at the time.

The second issue, which appeared 10 years later in 1952, contained the first research papers (in English, French, and German) by the Istanbul faculty, as well as his now trained students. Peters' own contributions include an article on the pragmatist philosopher John Dewey (1859–1952), who was one of the first to be invited to Turkey to evaluate the educational system (W. Peters, 1952a). More important is his key study, the *Intelligence Testing of a Thousand Turkish Children* written up in 1943 (W. Peters, 1952b). Between 1938 and 1943, Peters had undertaken a series of comparative studies of Turkish school children (age, gender, education, social level, city, and village). Based on the results, using the Terman's "Stanford Revision" of Binet and Simon's intelligence tests (see Figs. 9 and 10), Peters made a cultural comparison between the American

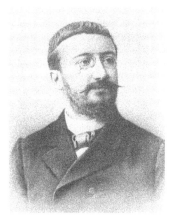

Figure 9. Alfred Binet (1857–1911).

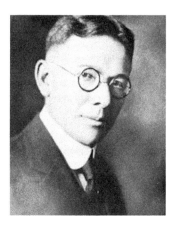

Figure 10. Lewis Madison Terman (1877–1956).

and Turkish children. Peters consistently found a correlation between the performance levels on the tests and the social and educational backgrounds. In a period of widely used IQ tests, and the eugenic emphasis on the heritability of psychological characteristics and social behavior (Gould, 1981; Tan, 1972), Peters stands out in considering the influence of social environment and educational background on what is inherited. To what extent he was influenced by his "observational work" at a time when traditional methods were being questioned at the Child Guidance Clinic in Britain also needs to be investigated. His publications from Istanbul University reflect a new direction (Peters, 1938–1944; 1952, 1956) in the areas of his former research interests. Being in Turkey appears to have provided him with an opportunity to turn from individual differences in psychology to consider cultural comparisons (Turkish, American, and middle European children) which may not have occurred had he remained at Jena.

Peters appears to have succeeded in building up an Institute of Experimental Psychology, paving the way for its independence from both philosophy and pedagogy (Toğrol, 1987). Such tangible achievements were not without a personal toll — fighting with the administration at every turn for space, funds, staff, and equipment. The Turkish faculty who had different orientations in psychology, were not persuaded by the importance or the practical application of experimental psychology. Others, with the increasing nationalist influences resented the presence of a "foreigner" (Riesman, 2006, p. 274) (see Figs. 11 and 12).

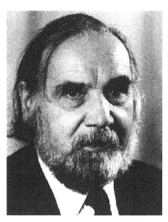

Figure 11. Wofgang Metzger (1899–1979).

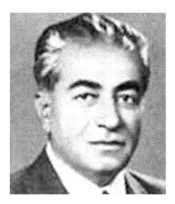

Figure 12. Muemtaz Turhan (1904–1969).

Peters' assistant and younger colleague, the Turkish psychologist Muemtaz Turhan (1908–1969) is singled out as the only exception to Peters' negative view of his colleagues.[19] Turhan was trained in Germany in experimental psychology and gestalt theory, under Wolfgang Metzger (1899–1979) at Frankfurt am Main, with a second PhD (1944) at Cambridge under Frederick Bartlett (1886–1969). The latter subsequently led to Peters' promotion to full professorship, even in the face of administrative obstacles. Turhan was a strong ally in this respect and translated many of Peters' lectures and articles. In return, it was upon Peters' emphatic recommendation that Turhan could receive the chair of the institute after Peters' own retirement.

In 1952, Peters resigned after 16 years in Turkey, when he returned to Germany, to the University of Wuerzburg as an emeritus professor at the age of 82. He remained there until his death in 1963, while rejecting the offer of reparation from the University of Jena that had previously dismissed him in 1933 (Holzapfel, 2001). The circumstances of his departure are complex and reflect the changes in the political and social climate of the postwar period. It is in part due to a legal detail of his contractual agreement concerning his leave of absence for surgery in Germany (Toğrol, 1983). The university committee set up to investigate the grounds for extending Peters' stay ended with a negative vote despite the efforts of supporting faculty and gave the government the needed excuse not to cover his medical expenses incurred in Germany. It was argued that Peters had failed to fulfill his contractual obligations. In particular, he had not learned Turkish, nor published any textbook for the use of the students, although it was

---

[19]His former student, who went on to Stanford and Cambridge for her training in psychology, recalls that "Peters was quite advanced in years, but an extremely intelligent and knowledgeable scientist; somewhat broken down and embittered by the experiences of his life. From time to time he would open up, and relate rather negative anecdotes about various colleagues. In all these conversations, however, the single exception for whom he could not find adequate words of praise, was M. Turhan, who was away in England at the time, completing his second PhD. Only those who knew Peters would appreciate the significance of such praise coming from him" (Toğrol, 1987; author's translation).

actually available in manuscript form and ready to go into print. He was further said to be unapproachable and far too demanding in his expectations of the students.[20] As his medical coverage only applied to injury within Turkey and not outside, he could not be reimbursed. He had taken a leave of absence without pay. Peters had no choice but to tender his resignation (Batur, 2005).

The grounds for Peters' departure raise questions. Did the government genuinely find that Peters did not adequately fulfill his contractual obligations to the state, or had he outlived his usefulness because of his age? To what extent was the decision a reflection of the changes in the political and social climate of the post-war period? Peters was not the only foreign academic to lose his position on a legal point. Part of the proffered explanations relate to the serious economic difficulties of the Turkish Government.[21] Despite genuine attempts in some cases, they lacked the funds to provide for the retirement of the émigré academics (Shaw, 2002).[22] Peters had survived the consequences of the shift of the Turkish foreign policy from being "neutral" to declaring war on Germany just before the end of the war. All the émigrés then found themselves citizens of an enemy country with the prospect of being prisoners of war, becoming stateless, or applying for Turkish citizenship. With the last option they were protected by the Turkish government (Konuk, 2010). Most of the emigration to the United States took place during that period (Reisman, 2008). A significant factor in Peters' situation was also the waning of the German and the rising of the American influence after the war that affected psychology (Vassaf, 1987; McKinney, 1960).

In Turkey, Peters had a new stability in contrast to his stay in Britain. He had been able to bring his whole family from Vienna shortly after his arrival. He not only kept the same academic appointment as chair, but was also promoted to the directorship of the Institute of Pedagogy and Psychology (see Fig. 13), where he could use his expertise and experience in building up experimental psychology as an independent discipline. Furthermore, he applied his pioneering work in IQ testing of children and adolescents to Turkish culture. In this way, he was able to continue and extend his original concern with the nature-nurture question, gaining evidence that reinforced his conviction of the influence of environmental factors on heredity.

In addition to job security, Peters had a salary that was higher than that of his Turkish colleagues, as was the case for all German academics. Due to inflation, however, it became

---

[20]None of the reasons were based on anti-Semitism or pertained to Peters' being Jewish. The émigré academics were perceived as "foreign guests" and "exemplary Europeans" and were not categorized as Jews (Konuk, 2012, pp. 121–150). The rise of anti-Jewish developments in Turkey in the 1930s and 1940s have been attributed to nationalist and Turkification policies. They were distinguished from the European anti-Semitism (see Çağatay 2006).

[21]To raise the desperately needed funds is put forth as one of the major reasons for the tax on minorities who constituted the wealthy middle class. The indiscriminate application across the board without consideration of the level of income led to the injustice with tragic conse-quences (Shaw, 2002).

[22]The experiences were complex. The memoirs relate both positive and negative reminisces and the gap between their expectations and the reality of with what they had to deal. The majority left after the war for the United States. Some stayed on and were buried in Istanbul, or given Turkish citizenship, and some would have liked to stay on but left for various reasons for the United States, including university education for their children (see Konuk, 2012; Widmann, 1973).

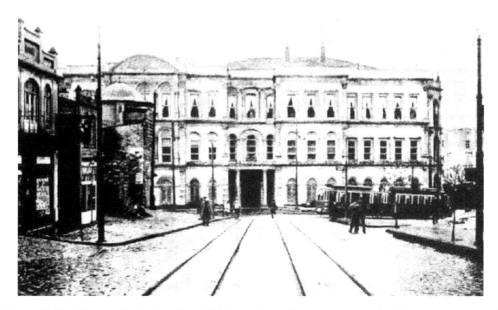

Figure 13. The Zeynep Hanim Mansion which housed the Faculty of Letters, including the Institute of Pedagogy and Experimental Psychology. The inadequacy of space was a major problem.

increasingly inadequate through the years and resulted in economic hardships among the émigrés. To claim the retroactive pension rights offered by Germany became a contributing factor in their return (Doelen, 2010; Bahar, 2010).

Muzafer Sherif (1906–1988) in Turkey: Another variation on the theme

In 1933, when the secular Turkish Republic offered 30 German-speaking academics and professionals, expelled by the Nazis, positions at Istanbul University, 87 of its own academics were dismissed from their university posts (ostensibly for obstructing government reform policies) to make room for the "foreign" professors (Doelen, 1999, pp. 237–239).

In the invitations no discrimination was made as to whether they were Jewish, communist, homosexual, or anti-Nazi activist and political dissidents. The selection criteria were based on their professional expertise and reputation as emissaries of European and Western knowledge. As such, they were the essential cogs in the wheel of university and cultural reform that was centralized by the state.

During this period there is no evidence that the German émigré scholars were facing any racial or political discrimination in Turkey. They remained, on the whole, like Wilhelm Peters, as "foreign guests," under state protection. Within a decade, Turkish academics and professionals were being dismissed from their positions or imprisoned for antigovernment (i.e., antifascist) activities and as communists with the change in foreign policy concerning the Soviet Union. At the same time, the rising pan-Turkist and nationalist political movements were being influenced by the imported German racial views.

111

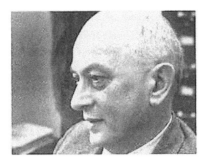

Figure 14. Muzafer Sherif (c. 1946).

A passionate intellectual

The country that provided a safe haven to German-speaking émigrés, where they survived the war, was ironically creating conditions that forced its own academics into exile. This is exemplified by Wilhelm Peters' younger contemporary, Muzafer Sherif (see Fig. 14), also a psychologist, at the University of Ankara, who for political reasons had to "escape" to the United States. Sherif's case extends the subject beyond that of Nazi Germany, and the German-speaking academics, into the broader interrelated phenomena of other exiled scientists in the twentieth century. It serves to demonstrate as well as provide significant insights into the complexity of issues behind the "brain drain–brain gain" equation, going beyond a specific place in time (Medawar & Pyke, 2001, p. 7).

When Peters arrived at Istanbul University, Sherif had just been appointed assistant professor at Gazi Institute in Ankara. Sherif had a thoroughly American education, starting with a BA in 1927 at the American International College in Izmir, set up by the congregational missionaries. After obtaining a Masters in 1929 at the *Daruelfuenun* — which was dissolved to become the University of Istanbul in 1933 — he had gone to Harvard for graduate studies from 1929 to 1932 on a government scholarship, earning a second MA in 1932. After a two-year interval in Turkey, he then completed his PhD at Columbia University (1934–1935) under Gardner Murphy (1895–1979) and became well known with the publication of his dissertation the *Psychology of Social Norms* (1936) (Harvey, 1989). He spent the period of the Second World War between 1939 and 1945 in Ankara.

Applying psychology — The use of intelligence quotient tests

Peters, despite his comprehensive background in experimental psychology, was involved in applied educational psychology. Sherif, on the other hand, regarded himself as a basic scientist, demonstrating what can be applied.

The early studies of Sherif with his students overlapped with those that Peters conducted with his students using IQ tests applied to Turkish children in cities and villages. At Ankara University, Sherif established a small research laboratory on social judgment from which he and his students translated several important texts on psychology into Turkish. These included the 1937 Stanford-Binet Test, along with chapters from Edwin

Garrigues Boring's (1886–1968) *History of Experimental Psychology* and Robert S. Woodworth's (1869–1962) *Contemporary Schools of Psychology*. They also conducted studies on adolescence and judgment scales of Turkish villagers who lived in varying degrees of isolation from modern technology. Sherif sought to identify the impact of technological and social reforms on villages that had previously been isolated. What concerned him was not applied research, but rather scientific investigation to understand (not why but how) and to demonstrate what can be applied. He wanted to provide answers to intergroup conflicts to combat the emergence of individualistic and reductionist explanations of human behavior (Sherif & Sargent, 1947).

Norm formation and social influence

While Peters was laying the foundation for an institute of experimental psychology, Sherif had already embarked on a series of creative studies in his small laboratory in Ankara. The result was his publication "*Some Social Factors in Perception,*" which used the autokinetic illusion phenomenon to look at people's judgments of the scale of apparent movement of a stationary pinpoint of light in an otherwise completely dark room. When individually estimating the apparent movements, the subjects tended to form their own personal reference scales. Yet, when brought together in a group, they tended to converge in their estimations. For Sherif, this "convergence" constituted the essence of "norm formation," one of the basic forms of social influence and conformity. The ideas and research from this experiment became the basis of his thesis and of his first classic text, the *Psychology of Social Norms* (Harvey, 1989).

Peters' intellectual background had molded his views and identity during the Weimar Period, the concept of general education ("*Bildung*") based on the enlightenment rationalism, had defined his identity as with the other émigrés (Mosse, 1983). Sherif's early years and personal experiences through the succession of major wars in Turkey had shaped his lifelong scientific concern. On his own admission, his research emerged from his experiences of war:

> As an adolescent with a great deal of curiosity about things, I saw the effects of war: families who lost their men, and dislocations of human beings. I saw hunger. I saw people killed on my side of national affiliation; I saw people killed on the other side.... In fact it was a miracle that I was not killed along with hundreds of other civilians who happened to be near one of the invasion points when Izmir [Smyrna] was occupied by an army, with the blessing of the victorious Western colonial powers at the end of WWI [First World War] .... I was profoundly affected as a young boy when I witnessed the serious business of transaction between human groups. It influenced me deeply to see each group with a selfless degree of comradeship within its bounds and a correspondingly intense degree of animosity, destructiveness, and vindictiveness toward the detested outgroups. Their behavior characterized compassion and prejudice, heights of self-sacrifice, and bestial destructiveness. At the early age, I decided to devote my life to studying and understanding the causes of these things. (Sherif, 1967, p. 9)

In moving towards social psychology, he was motivated by "intense intellectual curiosity and deeply felt compassion for human suffering" (Granberg & Sarup, 1988, p. 5). Thus, he focused his research to understand the influencing factors in attitude change, social judgment, and norm formation in intergroup relations (Harvey 1989). His *Realistic*

Conflict Theory (Sherif et al., 1961) validated his intergroup series of studies culminating in the now classic Robbers Cave Experiments (1954 and 1961) and "account[ing] for inner group conflict, negative prejudices, and stereotypes as a result of actual competition between groups for desired resources." It was followed by his unique approach to attitude change and social judgment theory (Harvey, 1989).

The dilemma of Nazi presence

Turkey's complex political "neutrality" and close (or "nonhostile") relations with Germany during the Second World War created an unusual situation where the émigré academics and the representatives of their Nazi persecutors were simultaneously present, working together at the same institution. An additional source of insecurity to encroaching German military expansion in Eastern Europe bordering on Turkey was the constant attempt of Nazi Germany to have faculty of its own recommendation appointed at Turkish Institutions. The Nazis sought to weaken the position of the émigré faculty since they exerted an "extraordinary influence on Turkish academic life" as the university as a whole had been "Judaized," undermining German influence with the Turkish government (Schwietering, 1961, p. 73). This was reported to Herbert Scurla (1905–1981), a writer and senior civil servant dispatched by the German Ministry of Science and Education, who prepared his own report on *The Activities of German Academics at Turkish Research Institutions*, based on his observations in Turkey in 1939 (Şen & Artunkal, 2008). It revealed that the Third Reich was monitoring the activities of the émigrés throughout the war in the Turkish Republic, using academics like the German Medievalist Henning Brinkmann (1901–2000) to report regularly to the Nazi officials in the embassy, to receive instructions from them, and to work in accordance with the Reich policies (Riesman, 2006; Konuk, 2012). This also reflects that the Turkish government had become more trusting of the exiled German scholars and rather suspicious of those who were appointed with the consent of the Nazi Government as working for German interests.[23]

The Turkish government countered such Nazi attempts to have faculty appointments of their supporters by inserting into the original 1933 faculty contracts a new additional clause, stating that no émigré faculty could be involved in political, economic, or commercial activities nor could act as an agent of propaganda for a foreign state or serve under any foreign institution or agency (Doelen, 2010). This is what Peters had signed.

Despite the strong opposition of the émigré faculty, including the negative vote of Peters, Henning Brinkmann was appointed in 1943, as the head of the German Language and Literature Department at Istanbul University for one year (Bahar, 2015). Brinkman, on the surface a German philologist and an ardent promoter of German classics with translations into Turkish, was a committed scholar in the service of the National Socialist state. Classified as

---

[23]This is also validated by the confidential report of the American Ambassador, J. van Antwerp McMurray (July 14, 1936): "It is understood that strong advocates and protectors of the professors exist in high circles in Ankara, and that any complaints which are made against them fall on deaf ears in the Capital" (see Riesman, 2006, p. 264).

"indispensable," he was an academic Nazi spy, expected to gather intelligence on all the activities of the *Philosophische Fakultaet* [The Faculty of Arts that included psychology]. While improving German-Turkish relations, he was to undermine the employment of "undesirable" Jewish faculty at the University of Istanbul (Correspondence with Herbert Scurla, of the Ministry of Education, May 27–June 5, 1944, as cited in Schwietering, 1999, pp. 74–76).

The presence of such faculty made life difficult for the anti-Nazi and Jewish academics. Peters had experienced the presence of racist Nazi faculty at his own institution at Jena. He had expressed his view of National Socialism in a series of lectures as a "Mass Mental epidemic" that may have hastened his dismissal from his position as an added factor to his being Jewish (Killy & Vierhaus, 1998). He continued to fight against the encroaching Nazi presence at Istanbul University by voting against Brinkmann when others abstained (Konuk, 2010).

Sherif had witnessed the spreading Nazi ideology, initially as an outside observer in Berlin then in his own country. On his way back to Turkey in 1932, he spent some time in Berlin to attend Koehler's lectures at Berlin University and also observed with "dismay and disgust" the effects of burgeoning Nazism. He became interested in the use of slogans by the National Socialists, that subsequently influenced the rising Fascism in Turkey. He had already conducted studies in "prestige-suggestion and stereotypes" (Sherif, 1935, pp. 370–375). He now turned to investigate the "psychology of slogans," and their role (Riesman, 2006b, pp. 273–275; Velten, 1998, p. 90) in attitude change, and the emergence of social norms (Sherif, 1937, pp. 450–461).

The Nazi presence was stronger in Ankara at the Gazi Institute and at the newly built Ankara University, where the persecuted and the persecutors were even working under the same roof (Velten, 1998; Riesman, 2006b; Bahar, 2015). Shortly after joining Ankara University (see Fig. 15), Sherif found himself in conflict not only with certain faculty and officials over their pro-Nazi attitudes but with the policies of the Turkish government that later had serious consequences for his personal safety. To combat its rising influence and the attempted application in Turkey of Nazi racial doctrine by showing its scientific absurdity, Sherif wrote the *Race Psychology* (*Irk*

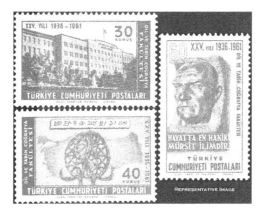

Figure 15. Commemorative stamp of the founding of Ankara University. At the entrance is Atatuerk's statement: "The true guide in life is knowledge."

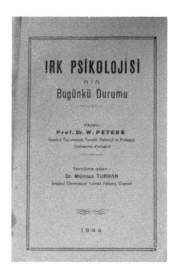

Figure 16. *The State of Race Psychology Today.* The title page of the Turkish translation of Wilhelm Peters' small book on "Race Psychology" (*Rassenpsychologie*, 1932) by Muemtaz Turhan with a foreword of its importance as a scientist's objective in publishing a sober exposition of a false doctrine, being politcially exploited, and to safeguard the reader from its dangerous ideological influences.

Psikolojisi) in 1943.[24] He stated, in response to public criticisms, that his book was just a summary of what was taught at Columbia University. Based mainly on Otto Klineberg's (1899–1992) *Race Differences* (see Figs. 16 and 17) and on Julian S. Huxley (1887–1975) and Alfred C. Haddon's (1855–1940) *We Europeans*, it was initially published as a series of essays, later as *The Changing World*, and in the anti-Nazi journal *Adımlar* [Steps] under his editorship (Granberg & Sarup, 1991). Sherif also took a stand against discrimination attempts by certain psychology faculty to fail a Jewish student, Rosette Avigdor (1923–2011), who subsequently completed her dissertation, *The Development of Stereotypes as a Result of Group Interaction* (obviously related to Sherif's theory) in 1952 at New York University (Granberg & Sarup, 1988).

In Ankara, Sherif had also become involved with communism. During the mass arrests of communists and antifascist faculty in 1944, Sherif was imprisoned, charged "for actions inimical to the national interest" (Trotter, 1985) and placed in solitary confinement for 40 days. His release was secured by the US Department of State at

---

[24]In 1944 Peters' work on race psychology, which was wriitten in 1932, was published in Turkish as the *State of Race Psychology Today*. In the Foreword, the importance of Peters' book, and the translator's objectives in publishing it are described in similar terms to those of Sherif (see Fig. 16). Responding to the public criticism of his *Irk Psikolojisi* [Race Psychology, 1943] by Mustafa Sekip Tunc (1886–1956), former chair of psychology at the University of Istanbul, Sherif stated: "Racial superiority is a foreign import. If it had not appeared in my country, 'Race Psychology' would not even have occurred to me. I am a social psychologist, as you know. . . If I have [with my book] succeeded in at least revealing the disgusting and evil true face of the advocacy of racial superiority, I would have served the intellectual life of my country. An advanced nation's views on human rights and values cannot be built on a falsehood" (author's translation).

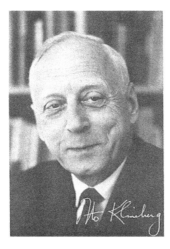

Figure 17. Otto Klineburg, Sherif's former teacher at the University of Columbia, whose *Race Differences* (1935) was a major source for Sherif's *Race Psychology*.

the instigation of influential Harvard alumni and colleagues, such as Hadley Cantril (1906–1969), Leonard W. Doob (1909–2000), Gardner Murphy (1895–1979), and Gordon Allport (1897–1967). He felt that he had in store an even harsher 27-year sentence and left for the United States in 1945 (Granberg & Sarup, 1988; Harvey, 1989). By 1951, as a result of the anticommunist purge, with many of Sherif's close friends and colleagues arrested or fled from the country and himself disowned by members of his family, Sherif's ties with Turkey had been irrevocably severed (Goezkan and Keith, 2015).

Sherif could neither return to Turkey nor take up US citizenship for fear of drawing attention to his communist associations, particularly during the political "witch hunt" by Senator Joseph McCarthy (1908–1957). In fact, Sherif was already on the suspect list of the Federal Bureau of Investigation (FBI).[25] Ironically, the FBI had also invented a new category specifically for the German-speaking émigrés, coining the term "communazis" (Stephan, 2000). Sherif himself remained stateless without a passport.

The personal price was heavy for both Sherif and Peters. Despite a brilliant career, honors and unflagging productivity,[26] Sherif suffered from manic depression in later years.

---

[25]Sherif was served with a warrant of arrest in deportation proceedings, charged with illegal extention of stay (FBI files, April 11, 1951). Released on conditional parole, his deportation was suspended (May 13, 1952) because of "serious economic detriment," and his 7 years of residence in the United States. See Batur S: Muzafer Sherif in FBI Files. In Goezkan AD, Keith DS (2015, chap. 4).

[26]His publications exceed 24 books and 60 articles. Much of his work, as a research professor of psychology at the University of Oklahoma, and later a distinguished professor of sociology at Pennsylvania State University, was jointly conducted with his wife, Carolyn (Koslin & Sills, 1979). In addition to his numerous honors between 1966–1978 for Distinguished Scientific Contribution in Psychology, he was the first ever to receive the Cooley-Mead Award for "substantial and lasting contributions to social psychology, particularly from a sociological perspective" (Harvey, 1989, p. 1329).

Whether or not this was associated with his war experiences or triggered by his solitary confinement for four months in a Turkish prison, or arrest in the United States for deportation, is not easy to determine. He attempted suicide on at least one occasion. His condition became even worse after his wife's death. Peters was already embittered and "broken down" by his experiences. In Turkey he had, nonetheless, laid the foundation for the first psychological laboratory to equip students with the tools and methods of experimental investigation, and a program of training in scientific research. The tangible outcome was 80 experimental studies, as well as doctoral theses (Toğrol, 1987). Despite his 16 years of service, the Turkish government refused to cover his medical expenses in Frankfurt, regarding it as "leave of absence without pay." Peters had become embittered by his experiences. As queried by one of Peters' former students, "How was it that a government so eager to welcome them in 1933 was so reluctant to keep them after their years of service?" (Toğrol, 1983, p. 6).

The Turkish government demanded Sherif's salary back for the two years of absence when he did not return to his post at Ankara University. In fact, he could not return. In addition to his previous involvement in the Turkish communist party, he faced a labor law according to which no "state employer" including the university faculty could hold a position if married to a foreigner. Sherif had married Carolyn Wood while at Princeton (see Fig. 18). He was dismissed from his position at Ankara University. In later years, he discouraged his two daughters from visiting Turkey even for a vacation as he was legally liable for the "salary debt" with cumulative interest over 40 years.

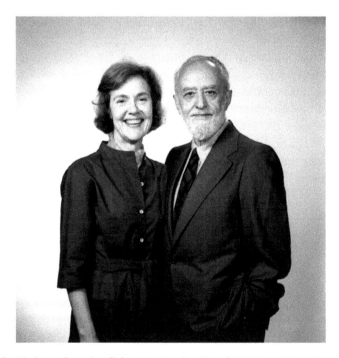

Figure 18. Sherif with his wife and collaborator Carolyn Wood (1922–1982), a distinguished psychologist in her own right.

Conclusion

This study reveals the complexity of issues behind the "brain-drain, brain gain" equation, at the professional, institutional, political, and cultural levels, as well as the personal costs. The cases of Wilhelm Peters and Muzafer Sherif encompass a broad canvas, involving Nazi Germany, Britain, Turkey, and the United States. This gives us a comparative view to identify the features that are specific to their individual experiences, and those that are shared, underlying translocation in science within the process of forced migration, regardless of a particular period, place, language, or culture.

References

Aldrich R (2002): *The Institute of Education 1902–2002: A Centenary History*. London, Institute of Education.

Anonymous (1936): East London Child Guidance Clinic (Lecture). *British Medical Journal* 1: 1123.

Ash M (1991): Central European émigré psychologists and psychoanalysts in the United Kingdom. In: Mosse WE, Carlebach J, Hirschfeld G, Newman A, Paucker A, eds., *Second Chance: Two Centuries of German-speaking Jews in the in the United Kingdom*. Tübingen, JCB. Mohr, pp. 101–121.

Ash M (2013): Weimar psychology: Holistic visions and trained Intuition. In: Gordon PE, McCormick JP, eds., *Weimar Thought. A Critical Companion*. Princeton, Princeton University Press, pp. 35–54.

Ash M (2015): *Universitaet – Politik – Gesellschaft. 650 Jahre Universitaet Wien – Aufbruch in das neue Jahrhundert*. Vienna, Vienna University Press.

Ash M, Soellner A, eds. (1996): *Forced Migration and Scientific Change: ÉmigréGerman-Speaking Scientists after 1933*. Cambridge, Cambridge University Press.

Bahar II (2010): German or Jewish, humanity or raison d'état: German scholars in Turkey, 1933–1952. *Shofar: An Interdisciplinary Journal of Jewish Studies* 29: 48–79.

Bahar II (2015): *Turkey and the Rescue of European Jews*. London, England, Routledge.

Batur S (2002): *Institutionalisierung der Psychologie an der Universtät Istanbul*. MA Thesis. The Faculty of Human and Social Sciences, The University of Vienna.

Batur S (2005): Psikoloji Tarihinde Koeken Mitosu ve Georg Anschuetz'uen Hikayesi. *Toplum ve Bilim* 102: 168–188.

Bentwich N (1936): *The Refugees from Germany April 1933 to December 1935*. London, George Allen & Unwin Ltd.

Bentwich N (1953): *The Rescue and Achievement of Refugee Scholars: The Story of Displaced Scholars and Scientists, 1933–1952*. The Hague, Netherlands, Martinus Nijhoff.

Brock AC, ed. (1992): *Internationalizing the History of Psychology*. New York, New York University Press.

Çağatay S (2006): *Islam, Secularism, and Nationalism in Modern Turkey*. New York, Routledge.

Carlebach J, Hirschfeld G, Newman A, Paucker A, eds. (1991): *Second Chance: Two Centuries of German-Speaking Jews in the United Kingdom*. Tuebingen, J. C. B. Mohr.

Doelen E (1999): Cumhuriyet'in onuncu yılında kurulmuş olan "İstanbul Ueniversitesi" ile Yueksek Ziraat Enstituesue'nuen kuruluşlarının ve akademik yapılarının karşılaştırılması. In: Toplu Bakış Uluslararası Kongresi Bildirileri, ed., *Bilanço 1923–1998: Tuerkiye Cumhuriyeti'nin 75 Yılına*. Istanbul, Cilt, pp. 235–249.

Doelen E (2007): Istanbul Darülfünunda ve Üniversitesinde Yabancı Öğretim Elemanları (Foreign Scholars in Istanbul Darülfünun and University). In: Aras NK, Doelen E, Bahadir, eds., *Türkiye'de Üniversite Anlayışının Gelişimi 1861–1961* (The Development of University Understanding in Turkey 1861–1961). Ankara, Türkiye Bilimler Akademisi Yayınları, p. 128. (See Appendix for Malche Report, pp. 352–399).

Doelen E (2010): Türkiye Üniversite Tarihi: 3. Darülfünun'dan Üniversiteye Geçiş (Tasfiye ve Yeni Kadrolar). *Istanbul Bilgi Üniversitesi Yayinlari* 277: 79–142; 445–469.

Ebbinghaus H (1908): *Psychology: An Elementary Textbook*. New York, Arno Press.

Eckardt G (2003): Der schwere Weg der Institutionalisierung – Wilhelm Peters. In: Eckard G, ed., *Psychologie vor Ort – ein Rueckblick auf vier Jahrhunderte. Die Entwicklung der Psychologie in Jena vom 16. bis 20. Jahrhundert*. Frankfurt am Main, Peter Lang, pp. 303–335.

Epstein A (1998): A lucky few: Refugees in Turkey. In: Berenbaum MA, Peck AJ, eds., *The Holocaust and History: The Known, The Unknown, The Disputed, and The Reexamined*. Washington DC, United States Holocaust Museum, pp. 536, 537.

Geuter U (1992): *The Professionalization of Psychology in Nazi Germany*, trans. Holmes RJ. Cambridge, England, Cambridge University Press.

Gould SJ (1981): *The Mismeasure of Man*. New York, W. W. Norton.

Goezkan AD, Keith DS (2015): *Norms, Groups, and Social Change: Muzafer Sherif's Psychology*. Transaction Publishers.

Granberg D, Sarup G (1988): *Social Judgement and Inergroup Relations: Essays in Honor of Muzafer Sherif*. New York, Springer.

Granberg, D, Sarup, G. (1991): Muzafer Sherif: Portrait of a passionate intellectual. In: Granberg D, Sarup G, eds., *Social Judgment and Intergroup Relations: Essays in Honor of Muzafer Sherif*. New York, Springer Verlag, pp. 3–54.

Harvey OJ (1989): Muzafer Sherif. *American Psychologist* 44: 1325–1326.

Holmes M (2010): Lives of emigrants: Duesseldorf—Berlin—Ankara—Washington: The Life of Edith Weigert (née Vowinckel) (1894–1982) (Translated by Cauleen S.). *Psychiatry* 73(1).

Holzapfel W (2001): Wilhelm Peters. In: Historische Kommission bei der Bayerischen Akademie der Wissenschaften, ed., *Neue Deutsche Biographie*. Berlin, Duncker & Humblot, Volume 20, p. 249.

Holzapfel W (2005): The relationship between theoretical memory psychology and art of memory: A historical analysis. *Passauer Schriften zur Psychologiegeschichte* 13: 105–114.

Jones E, Rahman S (2009): The Maudsley Hospital and the Rockefeller Foundation: The impact of philanthropy on research and training. *Journal of the History of Medicine & Allied Sciences* 63: 273–299.

Jones E, Rahman S, Woolven R (2007): The Maudsley Hospital: Design and strategic direction, 1923–1939. *Medical History* 51: 357–378.

Killy W, Vierhaus R, ed. (1998): Peters, Wilhelm. *Deutsche Biographische Enzyklopädie* 7: 617.

Konuk K (2010): *East West Mimesis: Auerbach in Turkey*. Stanford, Stanford University Press.

Konuk K (2012): *East-West Mimesis: Auerbach in Turkey*. Palo Alto, Stanford University Press.

Koslin B, Sills D, ed. (1979): *International Encyclopedia of the Social Sciences, Biographical Supplement*. New York, The Free Press.

Kravetz N (1993): *Displaced German Scholars: A Guide to Academics in Peril in Nazi Germany in the 1930s*. London, England, The Borgo Press.

Kreft G (2011): Dedicated to represent the true spirit of the German nation in the world. Philipp Schwartz (1894–1977), founder of the Notgemeinschaft. In: Marks S, Weindling P, Wintour L, eds., *In Defense of Learning. The Plight, Persecution and Placement of Academic Refugees 1933–1980s* (Proceedings of the British Academy, Vol. 169). Oxford University Press, pp. 127–142.

Kuruyazici N (1998): Farkli Bir Sürgün: 1933 Türkiye Üniversite Reform ve Alman Bilim Adamlari. *Alman Dili ve Edebiyatı Dergisi* 11: 37–50.

Mandler JM, Mandler G (1969): The diaspora of experimental psychology. The Gestaltists and others. In: Fleming D, Bailyn B, eds., *The Intellectual Migration, Europe and America, 1930–1960*. Cambridge, Harvard University Press, pp. 371–419.

Mazumdar P (2005): *Eugenics, Human Genetics, Human Failings: The Eugenics Society, Its Sources and Its Critics in Britain*. London, Routledge.

McKibbin R (1998): *Classes and Cultures in England (1918–1951)*. New York, Oxford University Press, pp. 254–256.

McKinney F (1960): Psychology in Turkey: Speculation concerning psychology's growth and area cultures. *American Psychologist* 15: 717–721.

Medawar J, Pyke D (2001): *Hitler's Gift: The True Story of the Scientists Expelled by the Nazi Regime.* New York, Arkade Publishing.

Mosse GL (1983): *German Jews Beyond Judaism.* Tel Aviv, Hebrew Union College Press.

Peters UH (1996): The emigration of German psychiatrists to Britain. In: Freeman H, Berrios GE, eds., *150 Years of British Psychiatry: The Aftermath.* London, England, Athlone, Volume II, pp. 565–580.

Peters W (1904): *Die Farbenwahrnehmung der Netzhautperipherie.* MD Dissertation, Wuerzburg, University of Wuerzburg.

Peters W (1932): Rassenpsychologie. In: Götze, Kretschmer, Peters, Weidenreich, eds., *Rasse u. Geist,* pp. 28–57.

Peters W (1940): İstanbul İlk Mekteplerinde Yapılan Test Araştırmaları. Birinci Rapor. *Pedagoji Enstituesue Psikoloji ve Pedagoji Çalışmaları* 1: 15–47.

Peters, W (1940b): Psikolojinin Bugünkü Durumu ve Antropoloji ile Münasebetleri. *Pedagoji Enstitüsü Psikoloji ve Pedagoji Çalışmaları* 1: 181–189.

Peters W (1943): Pedagoji Enstitüsü 1937–1943. *Pedagoji Enstitüsü Psikoloji ve Pedagoji Çalışmaları* 2: 1–9.

Peters W (1944): Öteki Mustafa Sekip. In: *Prof. Sekip Tunç Jübilesi.* Istanbul, pp. 55–57.

Peters W (1949): Memories of Ernst von Aster. *Felsefe Arkivi* 2: 19–36.

Peters W (1952a): Bin Tuerk Çocuğu Uezerinde Yapılan Zeka Testi Araştırmaları. *Pedagoji Enstituesue Psikoloji ve Pedagoji Çalışmaları* 2: 92–102.

Peters W (1952b): John Dewey als Psycholog und Philosoph. *Studies in Psychology and Pedagogy from the Institute of Pedagogy, University of Istanbul* 11: 183–192.

Reisman A (2006, November 20): What a freshly discovered Einstein letter says about Turkey today. *History News Network,* p. 1.

Reisman A (2006b): *Turkey's Modernization, Refugees from Nazism and Atatürk's Vision.* Washington, DC, New Academic Publishing.

Reisman A (2008): They helped modernize Turkey's medical education and practice: refugees from Nazism 1933–1945. *Gesnerus* 65: 56–85.

Reisman A (2009): *Shoah: Turkey, the US and the UK.* New York, New Academia Publishing.

Schwartz P (1995): *Notgemeinschaft. Zur Emigration deutscher Wissenschaftler in die Tuerkei,* ed. Peukert H. Metropolis, Marburg.

Schwietering J (1961): *Philologische Schriften,* ed. Ohly F, Wehrli M. Munich, Boehlau.

Schwietering J (1993): Hennig Brinkmann– Scholar, spy. In Hutton C, ed., *Linguistics and the Third Reich: Mother-Tongue, Fascism, Race and the Science of Language.* Routledge, pp. 74–77.

Şen F, Artunkal F (2008): *Ayyildiz Altinda Sürgün: Herbert Scurla'nin Nasyonal Sosyalism Döneminde Türkiye'de çalışan Alman Bilim Adamları Hakkında Yazdığı Rapor.* (Exile Under the Crescent and Star: Herbert Scurla's Report on the German Scholars Working in Turkey During the Period of the National Socialism). Günizi Yayıncılık.

Shaw SJ (2002): Roads East: Turkey and the Jews of Europe during World War II. In: Levy A, ed., *Jews, Turks, Ottoman: A Shared History Fifteenth through the Twentieth Century.* Syracuse, Syracuse University Press, pp. 246–260.

Sherif M (1935): A study of some social factors in perception. *Archives of Psychology* 27: 17–22.

Sherif M (1937): The psychology of slogans. *Journal of Abnormal and Social Psychology* 32: 450–461.

Sherif M (1943): *Irk Psikolojisi.* Istanbul, Universite Kitaberi.

Sherif M (1967): *Social Interaction: Process and Products.* Chicago, Aldine Publishing.

Sherif M, Harvey OJ, White BJ, Hood W, Sherif CW (1961): *Intergroup Conflict and Cooperation: The Robbers Cave Experiment.* Norman, OK, The University Book Exchange.

Sherif M, Sargent SS (1947): Ego-involvement and the mass media. *Social Issues* 3: 8–16.

Stephan A (2000): Communazis. In: *FBI Surveillance of German Émigré Writers,* trans. Van Heurck J. London, England, Yale University Press.

Tan H (1972): Development of psychology and mental testing in Turkey. In: Cronbach LJ, Drenth PJ, eds., *Mental Tests and Cultural Adaptation.* The Hague, Mouton, pp. 3–12.

Toğrol B (1983): Turkiye'de psikolojinin gelisim ve tarihcesi: Istanbul Universitesi. In: Bilgin I, ed., *Ulusal Psikoloji Kongresi.* Izmir, Ege Universitesi Edebiyat Fakultesi Yayinlari, pp. 82–91.

Toğrol B (1987): History of Turkish psychology. *Tecrübi Psikoloji Çalışmaları* 15: 1–7.

Trotter RS (1985, September): Muzafer Sherif: A life of conflict. *Psychology Today*, no page number.

Vassaf GYH (1987): Turkey. In: Gilgren AR, Gilgen C, eds., *International Handbook of Psychology*. Westport, Greenwood, pp. 3–12.

Velten K (1998): *Die Emigration deutscher Wissenschaftler in die Türkei 1933-1945*. University of Hamburg (Magister arbeit).

Weiss V (1980): Zum Gedenken an den 100: Geburtstag des Psychologen Wilhelm Peters. *Biologische Rundschau* 18: 295–300.

Widmann H (1973): *Die deutschprachige akademische Emigration in the Tuerkei nach 1933*. Bern, Frankfurt am Main, Herbert & Peter.

Eugenics ideals, racial hygiene, and the emigration process of German-American neurogeneticist Franz Josef Kallmann (1897–1965)

Stephen Pow and Frank W. Stahnisch

ABSTRACT

Biological psychiatry in the early twentieth century was based on interrelated disciplines, such as neurology and experimental biology. Neuropsychiatrist Franz Josef Kallmann (1897–1965) was a product of this interdisciplinary background who showed an ability to adapt to different scientific contexts, first in the field of neuromorphology in Berlin, and later in New York. Nonetheless, having innovative ideas, as Kallmann did, could be an ambiguous advantage, since they could lead to incommensurable scientific views and marginalization in existing research programs. Kallmann followed his Dr. Med. degree (1919) with training periods at the Charité Medical School in Berlin under psychiatrist Karl Bonhoeffer (1868–1948). Subsequently, he collaborated with Ernst Ruedin (1874–1952), investigating sibling inheritance of schizophrenia and becoming a protagonist of genetic research on psychiatric conditions. In 1936, Kallmann was forced to immigrate to the USA where he published *The Genetics of Schizophrenia* (1938), based on data he had gathered from the district pathological institutes of Berlin's public health department. Kallmann resumed his role as an international player in biological psychiatry and genetics, becoming president (1952) of the American Society of Human Genetics and Director of the New York State Psychiatric Institute in 1955. While his work was well received by geneticists, the idea of genetic differences barely took hold in American psychiatry, largely because of émigré psychoanalysts who dominated American clinical psychiatry until the 1960s and established a philosophical direction in which genetics played no significant role, being regarded as dangerous in light of Nazi medical atrocities. After all, medical scientists in Nazi Germany had been among the social protagonists of racial hygiene which, under the aegis of Nazi philosophies, replaced medical genetics as the basis for the ideals and application of eugenics.

Introduction

Beyond the obvious advantage of providing access to a plenitude of individual neuroscientists' biographies and institutional-clinical histories, the "artificial" situation of the massive exodus of scientists and physicians from the German-speaking countries also offers unique insights into the contingencies, contexts, and individual structures of knowledge transfer in neurogenetics and biological psychiatry (Ash & Soellner, 1996, pp. 10–15). The interests of this article are primarily related to how the process of forced migration influenced the cultural aspects of scientific and professional dynamics, as these pertain to interdisciplinary advances in biological psychiatry and clinical neuroscience since the middle of the twentieth century. It is clear that research into mental illness and neurological clinical care in North America and in the German-speaking countries changed significantly in twentieth-century biomedicine after the expulsion of so many émigré psychiatrists and neuroscientists (Magoun, 2002, pp. 165–240). A look at some of these early psychiatric and neuroscientific researchers allows us intriguing insights into the actual production of knowledge in the life sciences. Rather than seeing the phenomenon merely in terms of the escape of large numbers of émigrés to the United States and Canada, it can also be regarded as the unfolding of interactions between many knowledge groups. Refugee physicians and researchers introduced useful scientific directions, which differed from the traditional disciplinary methodologies, while establishing new and encompassing educational and training programs.

Individual neuroscientists, such as the Breslau neurological and psychiatric geneticist Franz Josef Kallmann (1897–1965), or local scientific milieus, for example, the specific working conditions he encountered at the Psychiatry Department at Columbia University's Medical School where psychoanalysis was predominant,[1] had decisive impacts on the future development of the neurosciences at large. This article on Franz Josef Kallmann's forced migration and medical career, as neurogeneticist, biological psychiatrist, and early epidemiologist, intersects well with a recent and larger historical research project that the corresponding author has begun over the past several years (e.g., Stahnisch, 2009). The latter has been attempting to investigate the emerging and coevolving neuroscience centers at the beginning of the twentieth century as places that brought together methods, practices, and approaches from the previously distinct clinical and research fields of neurology, anatomy, pathology, and especially brain psychiatry (today better known as biological psychiatry), as they were understood roughly a century ago (cf. Stahnisch, 2016a, pp. 25–30). The focus of our coauthored article for this Special Issue of the *Journal of the History of the Neurosciences* relates to particular developments in basic neuroscience that we refer to as the "neuromorphological sciences" — *avant la lettre* (i.e., before the term of the "neurosciences" was coined in the early 1960s; Pickenhain, 2002, p. 241f.) — and that strongly influenced the many émigré psychiatrists and neurologists who were affected by the process of forced migration in central Europe during the 1930s and 1940s (Stahnisch, 2010). The clinical fields of neurology and (brain) psychiatry come into the picture here, insofar as individual researchers and physicians were often actively trained in the basic neurosciences — in the German-speaking field of *Nervenheilkunde*[2] or took thematic problems from the clinical and public health side and integrated them into their research programs (Koehler & Stahnisch, 2014, pp. 1–4). In general then, we want to locate this process in the historical prelude to the development of the neurosciences as an interdisciplinary field in North America, that is, during the Second World

---

[1] Communication of the former Stephen and Suzanne Weiss Dean of the Cornell Medical School, New York City, Robert Michels (b. 1936) on September 5, 2012 with the corresponding author (F.W.S.).
[2] See also Holdorff (2016) in this special issue.

War and during the crucial postwar period of the 1950s and 1960s. The overall trends in the field are well illustrated by focusing on the process of forced migration and on a particular individual researcher who was affected by these historical events (see Roelcke, 2007, pp. 173–190).

The driving assumption underlying this article is that the first four decades of the twentieth century witnessed the emergence of new and distinct cultures of experimental neurology, neuroanatomy, and clinical brain psychiatry. These could be characterized as being proto-interdisciplinary and organized along the new lines of group research — *Gemeinschaftsarbeiten* in the terminology of the German Research Council (*Deutsche Forschungsgemeinschaft*), which had used such working arrangements since the 1920s.[3] They were early forms of big (neuro)science, which included the use of large funds, and they were attempting an integration of formerly disciplinary-bound knowledge spheres (Rose & Abi-Rached, 2013, pp. 1–24). These cultures likewise served as important research bases for innovative approaches in the laboratory investigation of the central nervous system (e.g., regenerative concepts or cortical brain-mapping projects), while also becoming hubs of new research trends in clinical neurology and psychiatry (Stahnisch, 2016b, pp. 1–3). This was a very important development in itself, as the changes in the early decades of the twentieth century not only led to important transformations on the organizational level in brain research but were necessary conditions, if the production of new forms of knowledge was to become possible at all.

Based on an influential interpretation by the Heidelberg and Berlin psychiatrist and neurologist, or *Nervenarzt*, Wilhelm Griesinger (1817–1868) — who stated that "all forms of mental disease are in fact diseases of the brain" (1867, p. 113) — early biological psychiatric research during the first half of the twentieth century was based in a number of interrelated disciplines, such as neurology, neuropathology, and areas of clinical psychology (Engstrom, 2003, pp. 51–55). The German-American psychiatric geneticist Franz Josef Kallmann is a very good, and also instructive, example of a highly innovative and multi-dimensional researcher from clinical neuroscience, who functioned exceptionally well in both scientific cultures — early in the field of neuropathology in Germany, as well as during his forced exile on the other side of the Atlantic — despite the marked differences in the contexts of his scientific pursuit between Berlin and New York (Mildenberger, 2002, pp. 183–200). Possessing innovative ideas, however, could be an ambiguous advantage for émigré neuroscientists, who were forced to leave Germany, Austria, and other countries of central Europe that were occupied before and during the course of the Second World War, since such ideas could easily lead to clashing scientific views. In some cases, they could result in the newcomer being sidelined in existing clinical or basic research programs (Born, 2011, pp. 79–83).

In this article, we will first introduce Kallmann's own development as a scientist and neuropsychiatrist, specifically in Munich and Berlin. Second, we will describe his later flight from Nazi Germany a few years before the outbreak of the Second World War and his adjustment to the American research and psychiatric context. Finally, we will assess the process of his adaptation to North American neuroscience and some of the constraints

---

[3]Notgemeinschaft/Deutsche Forschungsgemeinschaft, Praesidium Minutes (no day given, 1920), Bundesarchiv Koblenz, Germany, Collections on the *Deutsche Forschungsgemeinschaft* R 73/69/p. 63.

and resistance he encountered as a leading pioneer of genetic psychiatry and neurology in the United States of America.

Franz Josef Kallmann's early career in Germany

The continuing changes in the political and organizational frameworks of the German-speaking medical and health care system from the Weimar Republic to the seizing of power of the Nazi government in 1933 (Weindling, 1989, pp. 441–488) had a discernable influence on the Berlin-based psychiatric geneticist Franz Josef Kallmann. Yet, unlike many of his scientific peers, Kallmann can be viewed as an example from biological psychiatry of an individual researcher transitioning seamlessly in both political and cultural systems of the Weimar Republic and Nazi Germany (Benbassat, 2016, p. 1). Nazi laws and attitudes regarding his own Jewish ancestry eventually made continued residence and any sort of productive work in his homeland something of an impossibility, so that he ultimately took part in the large-scale pattern of emigration from Germany to North America in 1936 (Peters, 1996). What is truly remarkable, however, is that this by no means ended his close collaboration and research sharing with his colleagues who remained in Nazi Germany. Moreover, Kallmann once again transitioned successfully, this time into the American biological psychiatry milieu, so that rather than being sidelined like many of his colleagues who struggled with, for instance, the process of acculturation, he had a fruitful career in the United States and his contributions were widely recognized there, at least in the field of human genetics and biological psychiatry. His example testifies to the fact that research in the wider biomedical and health care area had already assumed a very important international and cosmopolitan character by the 1930s and 1940s, bringing together researchers and trainees from both sides of the Atlantic.

Franz Josef Kallmann (see Fig. 1) was born in 1897 near Breslau (modern-day Wrocław in Poland), which was then part of the Prussian province of Lower Silesia. The son of Marie Kallmann (1874–1942, née Mordze/Modrey) and Bruno Kallmann (1861–1941) (Cottebrune, 2009, pp. 296–300), his father was a trained surgeon who worked as general practitioner in his hometown. Born into the Jewish faith, Bruno had converted to Christianity in the latter half of the nineteenth century. Soon after Franz Josef Kallmann's graduation from high school (*Gymnasium*), he volunteered to join the German Army and took part in the counteroffensive against the advancing Russian troops on the Eastern Front in Prussia. Wounded on the battlefield multiple times, he returned to Breslau in 1916 and took up his medical studies (Mildenberger, 2002, p. 186). Already in the final stages of the First World War, Kallmann was receiving training at some of the German hotspots interested in the application of new experimental biological investigations of human genetics — namely, the Friedrich Wilhelms University of Bonn and the Friedrich Wilhelms University of Breslau. Franz Josef Kallmann received his *Dr. med.* degree from the latter institution in 1919 and began to practice as a clinical physician in psychiatry and neurology in various general hospitals of the city. During this time, he became quite interested in pursuing postgraduate scientific training, and, with this purpose in mind, he got into contact with Franz Alexander's (1891–1964) psychoanalytic institute in Berlin and the psychiatrist Karl Bonhoeffer at the Charité Hospital. It was with Bonhoeffer that he collaborated on

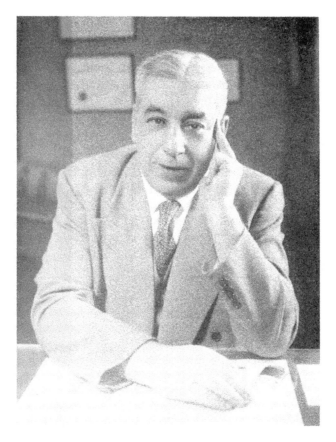

Figure 1. Franz Josef Kallmann, circa 1945. Image from the History of Medicine, National Library of Medicine, Bethseda, MD, USA.

questions of electrotherapy in neuropsychiatric patients with progressive paralysis (Marcuse & Kallmann, 1929), a group that included those he had first seen while working in the Breslau hospitals (Weber, 1993, p. 191).

At the University of Breslau, he had further shown some initial inclination toward the study of criminology, judging by his thesis, *Zufaellige Stichverletzungen als Todesursache* [Accidental Stab Wounds as Cause of Death] (Kallmann, 1921). Yet, it was neuropathology, particularly, that drew his scientific interest in the interdisciplinary and uniquely German field of *Nervenheilkunde*, that was characterized by an important overlap of approaches and methodologies with neurology, neuroanatomy, and neuropathology as they were practiced at the time (Stahnisch, 2014, pp. 25f.). He asked the eminent neuropathologist Hans Gerhard Creutzfeldt — of Creutzfeldt-Jacobs Disease fame — for advice and received an encouraging reply that he ought to pursue a career in neuropathology and brain psychiatry (Duckett & Stern, 1999, pp. 21–34). Creutzfeldt was also instrumental in bringing Kallmann into contact with Ernst Ruedin, the successor to psychopathologist Emil Kraepelin (1856–1926) in the directorship at the German Research Institute for Psychiatry in Munich, with whom he began to collaborate for a substantial period on investigations of sibling inheritance of schizophrenia (Roelcke, 2006, pp. 73–80).

From 1928 to 1935, Kallmann began to work as a neuropathologist in the large psychiatric asylum of Berlin-Herzberge on the eastern outskirts of the Prussian capital, where he continued to collect and amass considerable amounts of genetic data from the dissection "material" that he saw in the city pathological departments of Berlin. It was at the start of this period that he first became interested in the role of genetics in schizophrenia, a topic of research that was greatly facilitated by his collaboration with Ruedin in Munich. Between 1931 and 1935, Kallmann received several fellowships at the German Research Institute for Psychiatry (now the Max Planck Institute for Psychiatry), which housed more or less all of the leading figures of genetic psychiatry and, significantly, psychiatric twin studies, including Erik Essen-Moeller (1901–1992) and Hans Luxenburger (1894–1976) (Gershon, 1981, p. 273). Munich had become the center for this type of research ever since the founding of the German Research Institute for Psychiatry and its Genealogic-Demographic Department (*Genealogisch-Demographische Abteilung*) in 1918 after the end of the Great War.

Under the leadership of Ernst Ruedin, it provided the world's first institutional platform for the field of psychiatric genetics and scientific epidemiology. The years between the two world wars saw the Genealogic-Demographic Department grow in importance, garnering much international respect and often becoming a model for similar institutions elsewhere, such as at the University of Basel (Ritter & Roelcke, 2005, pp. 263–270). The close collaboration between the Genealogic-Demographic Department's protagonist Ernst Ruedin and the National Socialist regime, after its rise to power in 1933, was by no means an inhibiting factor for the growing worldwide recognition of the eugenic research conducted in Munich (Weber, 2000, pp. 234–250). Nonetheless, there were enormous transformations taking place in the general health care system of Nazi Germany. These have already been the subject of considerable research, looking at the legal pressures, changes in public health policies, and the reprehensible actions of many Nazi physicians in the eugenics and euthanasia programs that were being advanced since the start of the 1930s (Kater, 1992). Indicative of a formulation of eugenic policies predating the Nazi regime is a telling letter by Ernst Ruedin, written in early 1930, in which he was asking for financial research support and an alliance of psychiatric institutions, public health departments, and epidemiological research programs. Altogether, Ruedin and his collaborators in Munich aimed at:

> counting and identifying the mentally ill and handicapped as well as the respective disease prevalence in the individual regions of Germany, as we only know the numbers of the mentally and neurologically ill in the university and state hospitals and asylums, but do not know the prevalence of mental disease in the German provinces.[4]

As the political situation shifted, Kallmann's prolonged collaboration with the Munich institute also helped lay the groundwork for his becoming a pioneer in the field and protagonist of genetic research on psychiatric and neurodegenerative conditions. It further

---

[4]Ernst Ruedin, Letter (January 16, 1930) to Seine Excellenz Herrn Staatsminister Friedrich Schmidt-Ott (1860-1956), Historisches Archiv des Max-Planck-Instituts fuer Psychiatrie, Rockefeller Archive Center, International Finance Corporation (in alliance with the Rockefeller Foundation), Kaiser-Wilhelm-Institute for Brain Research, America's Great Depression Portfolio, pp. 45–46.

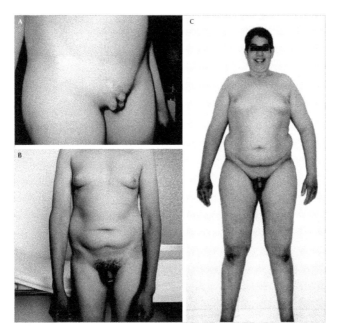

Figure 2. Phenotypical depiction of "Kallmann Syndrome" (Kallmann, Schoenfeld, & Barrera, 1943–1944).

belongs to this period that, in 1934, he described a genetic medical condition that later came to be associated with his name — the so-called "Kallmann Syndrome" (Dodé & Hardelin, 2010; see Fig. 2): It is a genetic condition that phenomenologically causes the failure to commence or the noncompletion of puberty and is characterized by hypogonadism, as well as a total lack of sense of smell (*anosmia*) or a greatly reduced sense of smell (*hyposmia*).

Though that genetic disorder bears Kallmann's name, the much more significant result of his work with the Munich German Research Institute for Psychiatry and its director Ernst Ruedin related to questions of the inheritance of schizophrenia in siblings. In that area, Kallmann had become one of the most well-known early researchers of genetic psychiatry on the international scale — as medical historian Florian Mildenberger from the University of Frankfurt/Oder has previously argued (Mildenberger, 2002, pp. 183–200).

For Kallmann, his role with the Munich researchers could only continue for a limited time following the Nazi seizure of power. Nazi leadership, of course, differed greatly from their predecessors in their ability to actually institute extreme policies aimed at racial hygiene, making use of the latest genetic research to justify these measures. Yet, it must be noted that Kallmann shared many of the prevalent views that even guided his mental health and genetic thinking in the postwar American public health context many years later:

It is rather unfortunate, therefore, that large segments of scientific workers, professional organizations and public health agencies are still inclined to cling to an attitude of timid inactivity, ideological compartmentalization or cynical indifference when confronted with some of the complexities of family relationships and population policies. If interdisciplinary approaches to the problems of mate selection, marital adjustment and parenthood are a necessity in modern societies, it is even more imperative that they should be plainly decodified and resolutely integrated. (Kallmann, 1952, p. 239)

While modern psychiatric geneticists have at times wished to downplay any affinity between the legitimate researchers in Munich and the Nazi ideologues, who eventually instituted eugenic policies, it is a difficult position to take based on the evidence (Joseph, 2006, pp. 142–143). Ruedin turned out to be an active protagonist of Nazi eugenics as were many of Kallmann's other colleagues. In this regard, Ruedin had to act as quite an ambivalent protégée to Kallmann, particularly when it became known that Kallmann was "half-Jewish" with respect to the Nuremberg Race Laws enacted by the Nazis in 1935 (Aly, 1994, pp. 26–29). In 1936, Ruedin was so worried that he might lose him — or better his exceptional research "know-how" — that he suggested Kallmann flee and find a new position in the United States from which they could still continue their mutual collaboration without Kallmann's life being put at risk by the Nazi government.

Kallmann's forced emigration to the United States and later career

It was not actually an easy decision for Kallmann to emigrate from Germany to the United States, particularly since he had been a German patriot since his days of military service during the First World War. While the Nuremberg Laws of 1935 had deemed him "half-Jewish," Kallmann himself did not identify along such racial or religious lines, and, when political pressure was exerted to end his work, he even relied on his colleagues in Munich to present his papers (Gershon, 1981, p. 273). He furthermore wholeheartedly approved of eugenics and the very restrictive medical programs in the Nazi public health service (Kallmann, 1945, pp. 522–524). In fact, he viewed them as rational and medically advanced and, thus, as part of a social progressivist program with which he himself associated the benefits of social psychiatry, psychiatric, and neurological genetics.[5] Kallmann's own personal risk to stay in Germany, and even more so the unknown future his parents faced in Breslau, finally led him to the difficult decision to emigrate (Rainer, 1972, p. 358f.). This was facilitated by letters of reference written November 21, 1936, by Dr. Karl Johann Petersen-Berstel (b. 1880?) from the Provincial Hospital and Nursing Home in Plagwitz near Leipzig to the German-American anthropologist Franz Boas (1858–1942) at Columbia University who was then in the role of president of the German-American League for Culture (*Deutsch-Amerikanischer Kulturverband*):

> Dr. Kallmann has been working at this institution since April 24, 1920. Since Dr. Kallmann possessed at the moment of his joining a certain preliminary education in psychiatry because of his work at the University Psychiatrical Clinic at Breslau, we soon could put him [in] charge of his own sick stations, under supervision of an older physician. [...] We got to know Dr. Kallmann as a young colleague, particularly qualified for the science of psychiatry, who is ambitious and industrious. We wish him all that is good for his future.[6]

---

[5]This seemingly incongruous situation is very similar to what we see in the recent historical research on émigré psychiatrists in Palestine, for example, by Israeli historian Rakefet Zalashik (2012).

[6]Franz Josef Kallmann, Letter to the Geman-American anthropologist Franz Boas at Columbia University (November 21, 1936) in his role as the president of the German-American League for Culture (Deutsch-Amerikanischer Kulturverband); Boas Collection of the Archives of the Library of Congress, Washington, DC, United States (professional transl./minor adjustment by authors) (LOC, Franz Boas Collection, 1936, Microfilm, Fond No. MSS60202).

Boas was very well connected and, as a member of the board of the Emergency Committee of German Displaced Scholars, stayed in contact with numerous physicians, scientists, and engineers, while trying to help place refugee academics in ongoing positions in the United States. To state that the process of emigration was simplistic for neurologists, psychiatrists, or any of their fellow exiles would be a gross exaggeration. Individuals like Kallmann rather found themselves in the foreign environment of North America, where they had to manage the new challenges of daily life, to support their families, to become relicensed and to try to achieve professional acceptance. They had to learn social and cultural codes, different mentalities, and "soft working skills" that were often learned the "hard way" (Rheinberger, 2005, pp. 187–197).[7] For many, it meant having to change research interests, so as to fit more closely with the acceptable clinical and scientific paradigms of the often hands-on, capitalist, and technophile North American society (Stahnisch, 2016b, p. 5). For Kallmann in particular, the challenges were quite severe. He barely spoke English upon his arrival in New York in the autumn of 1936. Social conventions, especially those in an academic setting, were strange to him and a serious issue of contention was his preference for genetic research over psychoanalysis (Kallmann, 1939). He initially worked in the psychology department of the New York State Psychiatric Institute for a small stipend, and his first attempts to return to genetic research were aided only by his wife, Helly (1899–1984) (Erlenmayer-Kimling et al., 1965, p. 123). She often took on the laborious data compilation and analysis work for him (Gershon, 1981, p. 274). A letter, written to anthropologist Franz Boas shortly after his arrival in North America, expresses what Kallmann must have hoped would make his past experience in Germany's genetic research programs an advantage rather than a liability in an American employment setting:

> Besides other scientific work in the realm of Clinical Psychiatry and cerebral anatomy (list is attached), I devoted myself since 1929 principally to research in hereditary psychiatry and hereditary biology and carried on an investigation of the hereditary genetic and fertility conditions within the circle of the various forms of schizophrenia in which investigation I was aided by the above mentioned clinics and the Berlin authorities and which in the meantime had been generally acknowledged by the competent scientific circles and particularly by the German scientists as being fundamental.[8]

In another even earlier letter to Boas, Kallmann describes his sense of upheaval while being careful to indicate his own distance from the alarming ideology and policy formulation that was taking place in the German psychiatry and neuropathology milieu from which he himself had scientifically emerged:

> I arrived here [in North America] with my wife 14 days ago and am trying to get back to normal both professionally and as a human being. As you can glean from the appended documents, I am a psychiatrist and neuropathologist by training, but I've been mainly concerned with psychiatric genetic research over the past years. And since, on the basis of my particular work and experiences, I believe I am capable and justified — as well as feeling

---

[7]Regarding an exploration of these cultural differences in émigré neurologists' and neuropathologists' working conditions in their home and new host countries, please refer to the Stahnisch (2016c) article in this special issue.

[8]Franz Josef Kallmann, Letter to Franz Boas at Columbia University (December 6, 1936); Boas Collection of the Archives of the Library of Congress, Washington, DC, United States (authors' translation) (LOC, Franz Boas Collection, 1936, Microfilm, Fond No. MSS60202).

obligated — to commence a battle against the pseudoscientific political theories in modern-day Germany, which I intend to rebut, I would appreciate it very much if you could offer me the kind opportunity for a personal meeting and exchange with you.[9]

We can see already in this letter the development of a narrative, which, if not fully accurate, was probably deemed by Kallmann to be indispensable if he was to have any hope of integration into the American psychiatric community. His "official biography," which came to be vociferously defended by some of his later students, was that, in the first years of the Third Reich, he had spoken out against Nazi laws calling for the "compulsory sterilization of psychotic patients," for which he was driven into exile. In fact, Mildenberger has demonstrated that, while he was in Germany, Kallmann called for an even more radical sterilization program for the mentally ill than that in place (Mildenberger, 2002, pp. 186–189).

Kallmann's intimation that his arrival in New York signaled a break with his former scientific practices, theories, and colleagues was expedient but events bear out that it was far from the truth. Despite what genuine resentments he felt toward his homeland, what is clear is that, from the mid-1930s, Kallmann brought the field of study, which he had put into practice in Munich, to the United States (Rainer, 1966, p. 413). His interests continued to mirror those of contemporary researchers in the Third Reich. During the same time period, when Ernst Ruedin at the German Research Institute for Psychiatry in Munich, Ottmar Freiherr von Verschuer (1896–1969) at the Berlin Kaiser Wilhelm Institute for Anthropology, Human Heredity and Eugenics, and the SS (Security Services) physician Josef Mengele (1911–1979) at the Institute for Hereditary Biology and Racial Hygiene at the University of Frankfurt began their twin studies in psychiatric asylums and later in concentration camps, such as Auschwitz (Weindling et al., 2016, p. 1f.), Kallmann himself embarked on his twin studies of schizophrenia and manic-depressive illness on the data of 700 siblings in various New York State hospitals with the support of the Department of Mental Hygiene (Kroener, 1998, pp. 32–35). For many years, these findings in conjunction with the former Berlin psychiatric data provided the major evidence for the influence of genetic factors in schizophrenic and manic-depressive illnesses a full generation before American and Danish adoption studies came to confirm these findings (Essen-Moeller, 1941, pp. 3–19; Slater, 1968, pp. 15–26).

The twin studies, which he had mainly conducted in Germany, led to the important publication of Kallmann's most well-known work only two years after his arrival in the United States. This was his hallmark study, *The Genetics of Schizophrenia: A Study of Heredity and Reproduction in the Families of 1,087 Schizophrenics* (1938a), which became the major reference publication for psychiatric and neurological twin studies and was a seminal textbook for the foundation of modern psychiatric epidemiology (Kaplan & Sadock, 1995, p. 1324). In fact, the work was based on the data he collected earlier from his time at Berlin–Herzberge and that he had brought with him on the steamship to Ellis Island, New York. It had been assembled from the Berlin district pathological departments of the city's public health department (Torrey & Yolken, 1966, pp. 105–106).[10] Based on 13,851 relatives of 1,087 patients admitted to Berlin hospitals over a decade, Kallmann's

---

[9]Karl Johann Petersen-Berstel, Letter to Franz Boas at Columbia University (October 26, 1936); Boas Collection of the Archives of the Library of Congress, Washington, DC, United States (authors' translation) (LOC, Franz Boas Collection, 1936, Microfilm, Fond No. MSS60202).
[10]See also Holdorff (2016) in this special issue.

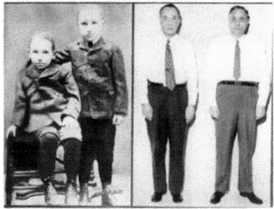

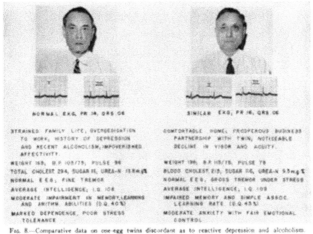

Figure 3. A prospective comparison of a twin couple, based on behavioral observations and physiological data collection from the 1940s. (Kallmann, 1956).

published research showed that siblings of schizophrenics have a 10 times increased risk for being diagnosed with the disease as well (e.g., see Fig. 3). The likelihood for other relatives of schizophrenics was only slightly higher than in the normal population — a conclusion he reiterated in his influential paper "The Genetics of Human Behavior" in the *American Journal of Psychiatry* (Kallmann, 1956, pp. 496–501). So, it could be said that Kallmann's initial work in the United States was the publication of his findings made in his early career on the other side of the Atlantic.

Moreover, he still held very close ties to his former colleagues and researchers, such as the Berlin psychiatrist Karl Bonhoeffer, Ernst Ruedin, and the Berlin psychologist Theodor Lange (b. 1891). This continued during the Nazi period, and long after Kallmann had assumed his new position within the New York State Psychiatric Institute.[11] These

---

[11]Collection on the Kaiser-Wilhelm-Institute for Psychiatry (also known as the German Research Institute of Psychiatry; Archives of the Max-Planck-Society [Harnack House], Berlin, Germany [fond no. Vc. Abt. Rev. 3. Nr. 15]).

relationships were lasting, and, with Kallmann's reputation as a formidable presence in biological psychiatry through his major publication in 1938, his views on the role of government policy regarding eugenics appear to have survived the transatlantic voyage as well:

> The danger of the development of new schizophrenic cases, arising from such unions, is so great that *there should be legal power to intervene*, in addition to the general eugenic program of the biological education of all adolescents, marriage counsel, obligatory health certificates for all couples applying for a marriage license, and the employment of birth control measures. (Kallmann, 1938b, p. 107)

Kallmann ran his genetics laboratory at the New York State Psychiatric Institute for more than two decades between 1938 and 1961, as he steadily regained his central role as a major international player in clinical psychiatric research and human genetics (Panse, 1966, pp. i–iv). He also managed to organize, despite obstacles, the first department of genetic research in the United States. His successful integration in North America was further emphasized when he became a cofounding member of the American Society of Human Genetics in 1948; and he later assumed his presidency (1952). The foundation of this society ultimately led to the planning of the Human Genome Project. Perhaps as the culmination of his career, he took on the directorship of the New York State Psychiatric Institute after 1955. During this period and until his death, Kallmann was financially supported by the National Institute of Mental Health (NIMH), based on his collaborative investigations with the Laboratory of Psychology (Slater, 1965, p. 1440).

It should not be imagined that Kallmann's gradual success in American medical and scientific communities was commensurate with his ability to adapt and take on the prevailing cultural attitudes toward eugenics and anything resembling racial hygiene. In fact, even in the postwar period, he remained quite outspoken about his positive views of "eugenics" as a foundational science area for a future biological psychiatry and the neurological assessment of inherited disorders. In fact, few years after the end of the Second World War, he asserted that the geneticist had a social obligation to pursue eugenics in his presidential speech, delivered at the fifth annual meeting of the American Society of Human Genetics at Cornell University (1952). The speech appeared as an article for the *American Journal of Human Genetics*, entitled "Human Genetics as a Science, a Profession, and as a Social-Minded Trend of Orientation" (Kallmann, 1952, pp. 237–245). For Kallmann, research on schizophrenia had convincingly established a genetic connection, which later studies were only to confirm. Though the Danish and American adoption studies swayed public opinion toward a genetic connection in schizophrenia only in the late 1960s (Essen-Moeller, 1941, pp. 3–19; Slater, 1968, pp. 15–26), Kallmann had arrived at such conclusions long before (Kallmann, 1950). Moreover, since he had observed genetic connections, it was his firm opinion that the aim of psychiatry in the field of schizophrenia had to be, primarily, a eugenic one:

> [A]s long as psychiatrists are satisfied by the theory that schizophrenia is only a psycho-pathological reaction which can be produced by unfavorable environment, illegitimacy, or psychosexual or other traumas, so long will it be impossible to make definite advance toward the eugenic goals of psychiatry in the field of schizophrenia. (Kallmann, 1938b, p. 105)

Thus it was that Kallmann continued to actively pursue a eugenic cause. He became the director of the American Eugenic Society (AES) in 1952 (Mehler, 1988, pp. 308) and, after a year, returned to that role from 1954 to 1965. A long-term member of this group was none other than Otmar Freiherr von Verscheuer, the aforementioned eugenics director at the Kaiser Wilhelm Institute for Anthropology, Human Heredity and Eugenics and a strong advocate for racial hygiene in the Nazi era. Like many of his colleagues, he had made the transition to becoming a legitimate genetics researcher who was unquestioned in the international sphere during the postwar era. Many networks remained in place through the twentieth century's upheavals.

Eugenics was of course not Kallmann's sole focus. He was fundamentally a physician and educator whose work inspired geneticists in training (Gershon, 1981, p. 273). A prolific writer, he wrote 176 papers and 49 books and pamphlets touching on subjects such as schizophrenia, tuberculosis, and genetic disorders. He was also involved in the development of family counseling, and, in 1955, he engaged in a pilot study to find better ways to provide counseling for deaf psychiatric patients, increasingly inspired by the growing trend of social psychiatry (Cottebrune, 2009, pp. 320–321). He died of cancer on May 12, 1965, at the same Columbia Medical Center where he had devoted roughly three decades to his scientific and clinical pursuits. His former student, John D. Rainer (1922–2000), remembered him as "a scientist in the broadest sense with a fertile imagination [...] a scanning interest in all of human activity [...] and the constant ability to frame richly suggestive hypotheses and to formulate careful research plans for their investigation" (Rainer, 1966, p. 413).

On the advantages and disadvantages of cutting-edge research as a refugee scientist

Since his arrival in the United States in 1936, Kallmann had fought an uphill battle for his acceptance into the North American scientific community, but ultimately he was able to establish himself as a leading researcher in the field of psychiatric genetics (Shorter, 2005, pp. 118–120). Interestingly enough, the fact that his type of research had been heavily supported by the National Socialist regime before was not an insurmountable barrier to his acceptance. At the New York State Psychiatric Institute — then an associated part of the Department of Psychiatry at Columbia University's Presbyterian Hospital ("The Old Presb")—he was able to continue his pioneering sibling studies (see Fig. 4). Eventually, he even became head of medical genetics at the Columbia–Presbyterian Medical Center and developed a full-scale research program, which he had early on envisioned in a letter to Franz Boas in 1936:

> The research [which I now intend to carry on] must be as representative and scientifically exact as possible and thus should fill a gap in our knowledge. It is hoped that this research will not only enable us to ascertain the cause for the origin of certain hereditary diseases, but also a way to prevent them. To carry on this research, a small special department is required at a psychiatric or genetic institute of first rank like for instance at the Psychiatric Clinic of Columbia University.[12]

Kallmann's work in New York included the examination of race-hygienic motifs, and he designed a research program that was directly based on concepts and methods from

---

[12]Franz Josef Kallmann, Letter to Franz Boas at Columbia University (December 6, 1936); Boas Collection of the Archives of the Library of Congress, Washington, DC, United States (authors' translation) (LOC, Franz Boas Collection, 1936, Microfilm, Fond No. MSS60202).

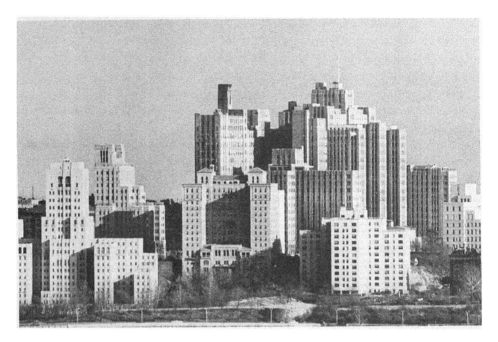

Figure 4. The Columbia-Presbyterian Medical Center (*Columbia University Bulletins of Information*, 1968). © Public Domain.

Ernst Ruedin's team of epidemiological researchers in Munich (Joseph & Wetzel, 2013, pp. 1–5). The only deviation from the original research, which he had practiced in Germany, was in terms of the use of eugenic prophylaxis in order to align his research to the context of North American democracy in the postwar era. However, the eugenic goal of elimination of certain categories of peoples remained unchanged — and Kallmann even continued to lecture on such negative eugenics methods even into the 1960s, for instance, at workshops of the National Institutes of Health in Bethesda, MD.[13]

Clearly, the political intentions of Nazism were very different from the mental health care system in the United States in the postwar period, but it is necessary to see the similarities in the scientific approaches in the medical and research landscapes on both sides of the Atlantic. Medical scientists were, in the pursuit of their research aims, among the protagonists and inventors of racial hygiene and broadened medical genetics, even if the idea of genetic differences in human behavior found little support among psychiatrists. It was exactly at this point in the mid-twentieth century, when there was uncertainty regarding the direction of future research, that the contributions of the National Institutes of Health (NIH) became vital for the advancement of interdisciplinary thought in the

---

[13]Clinical biochemist and later director of the History Office of the National Institutes of Health, Alan N. Schechter attended these sessions as a young National Institutes of Health Postdoctoral Fellow at the time. In a conversation with the corresponding author (Bethesda, MD, April 24, 2007), he remembered to have heard Kallmann actively presenting on "eugenics" in his lectures during the early 1960s. Apparently, Kallmann personally thought that the eugenics ideal would and should serve as the guiding principle of all modern genetic research, including psychiatric genetics approaches, without critically assessing the ethical digressions of the Nazi eugenics and euthanasia programs in this context.

growing field of biological psychiatry that Kallmann was helping to foster. The founding of the National Institutes of Health in 1948 and particularly the research conducted by the National Institute of Mental Health in the 1950s were landmark events, marking a pivotal phase in the formation of early neuroscience research activities when many émigré doctors and neuroscientists received relicensure and intended to resume professional work in medical research and clinical care in North American postwar neuroscience institutions (Pearle, 1984, pp. 112–137). This was undoubtedly an advantageous turn of events for Kallmann personally. When looking into the annual reports of the National Institute of Mental Health, it is possible to trace the financial support for his research program based on collaborative investigations with the Laboratory of Psychology in the intramural program for a period of nearly one and a half decades between 1952 and 1965 (Slater, 1965, p. 1440).

So there was a complex interplay, which yielded both advantages and disadvantages for Kallmann, who was receiving support from the National Institute of Mental Health while simultaneously struggling to find acceptance, or at least tolerance, from the wider discipline of psychiatry. As Eric Kandel (b. 1929), a fellow émigré psychiatrist, later reflected, the 1950s were a time when academic psychiatry willingly abandoned its roots in biology and evolved into "a psychoanalytically based and socially oriented discipline that was surprisingly unconcerned with the brain as an organ of mental activity" (Kandel, 1998, p. 457). Kallmann's speech as president of the American Society of Human Genetics in 1952, the same year that he started receiving National Institute of Mental Health funding, reflects the legitimate fear that transgressing the duality of mind and body would inevitably trigger hostility and stigma toward the geneticist:

> I was tempted for a short time to dwell on the need of giving priority, in man, to the mutative effects and selective values of *mental* traits, apt to be subject to the same genetic principles as demonstrated for scores of essential physical potentialities. However, such a topic of psychiatric coloring was certain to reopen the door to that hoax of dualistic setting, which contributed so heavily to a crippling division in other scientific disciplines. In fact, the urge to maintain a dichotomy of body and mind seemed almost as harmful as splitting a personality, and I soon remembered that psychiatrists were trained to cure schizophrenic phenomena rather than provoke them. (Kallmann, 1952, p. 239)

The dynamic of tension that persisted in those early years between biological psychiatrists and the psychoanalysts was echoed in the National Institute of Mental Health director's introduction, Dr. Seymour S. Kety (1915–2000), to the annual report of 1954, which clearly stated the widespread reluctance to accept genetic evidence as an integral part of biomedical knowledge in the psychiatric, and in the psychological or psychoanalytical communities, as well:

> As a result of the concern expressed by the National Advisory Mental Health Study Section over the failure of past research efforts to produce more definite results in relating the biological sciences to the field of mental health, a committee was established to determine the reasons for this failure and to search for means to stimulate better research in this area. [...] It was brought out that in some areas indefinite results have been due to failure to realize the complexity of the nervous system. The Committee also found that the most productive studies to date have been carried out on mental subjects, in which the imposed biological and psychological variables can be more adequately controlled. A continuing concern of the

Committee has been the biophobic and psychophobic attitudes of representatives of the behavioral and biological disciplines, respectively, and the problem of communication that exist between one field and another. (Kety, 1954, p. 3)

Thus, the story of Kallmann's emigration and adaptation in the United States reflects the intricate relationship between the new field of psychiatric genetics, eugenics, and public health politics in the Third Reich, as well as strategic research decisions taken by the directors of the individual National Institutes of Health on the western side of the Atlantic. We are constantly reminded of the ongoing influence that Nazi political and social developments had on these fields. Though Kallmann's work ended up being well received among American and international geneticists, the idea of genetic differences hardly caught on in contemporary psychiatry in the United States during his lifetime, as he himself lamented while reflecting on the 1950s psychiatric community's unwavering focus on environmental influences:

It is a plain but easily misjudged fact that in relation to human health and personality development, hereditary influences are thought of as static, while environmental influences are believed to be amenable to almost infinite manipulation. Actually, there is no single force in man's life and struggle for existence, which is more powerful, more dramatic or more inspiring than the one derived from the *dynamics of human heredity*. (Kallmann, 1952, p. 244)

The major reasons for this has already been intimated; as eminent historian of psychiatry Gerald N. Grob (2000, pp. 232–240) has pointed out, it was largely a result of the strong influence of a particular group of émigrés, the psychoanalysts, who came to dominate clinical psychiatry in the United States from the 1940s to the 1960s. The psychoanalysts established an important new cultural and philosophical trend, in which genetics played no significant role and was often regarded as a dangerous form of knowledge, after Nazi medical atrocities had been brought to light at the end of the Second World War (Grob, 1983, pp. 126–143). Indeed, that it took Kallmann a long time to establish the field of psychiatric eugenics in the United States can partially be explained by the predominance of psychoanalytic clinical research methods, which characterized the period and milieu in which he had reestablished himself. In the immediate postwar decades, the psychoanalytic clinicians and therapists showed a determination to give hereditary transmission short shrift. A few years before his death in 1965, Kallmann composed an autobiographical chapter that he entitled "That Rare Specimen — A Psychiatrist Concerned with Genetics" (unpublished), which alluded to the contemporary sense that no rapprochement would be forthcoming between clinical psychiatry and genetics (Kallmann, 1963). However, as John D. Rainer noted in a speech, upon the Stanley R. Dean Award being bestowed posthumously to Kallmann in 1966 for his contributions to schizophrenia research and the advancement of biological psychiatry, such a rapprochement was actually starting to take place, "sparked by the refinement of laboratory techniques as well as the detailed study of the differences among infants and children" besides Kallmann's own role in establishing interdisciplinary networks that encompassed geneticists, neurologists, pathologists, psychiatrists, and others (Rainer, 1966, p. 413).

Kallmann's example can thereby be interpreted as a double fracture of the historical events. Medical scientists and clinicians were among the social protagonists who pursued their research aims in a health care system framed by Nazi philosophies, and they were also among the major theorists of racial hygiene, which largely subsumed medical genetics as a scientific foundation for the ideals and applications of eugenics (Cornwall, 2003, pp. 71–90). Pursuing the goals of racial hygiene in the Third Reich, they had played a role in driving a large part of their Hippocratic brethren out of office and into exile. When the same neurologists and psychiatrists were, in turn, compelled to relocate or work in North America, diverging scientific traditions came to meet once again under changed scientific and hierarchical contexts in North American democratic societies (Davie & Koenig, 1949).

Discussion

When the National Socialist state was created in 1933, an exodus of the anti-Nazi elite began, including mostly Jewish physicians and scientists but also political opponents (communists and socialists), as well as researchers from abroad who did not intend to stay in Germany under such austere and depressing conditions (Medawar & Pyke, 2001, pp. 231–240). However, some researchers who were forced to leave Germany approved of Nazi eugenic politics, and these included Jewish physicians and scientists as well, as Rakefet Zalashik has intriguingly argued (Zalashik, 2012, pp. 33–39). One of them was the psychiatrist Franz Josef Kallmann, a researcher on schizophrenia and mental health disorders, who demanded an even more radical sterilization policy than the Nazis. He cooperated closely with the German Research Institute for Psychiatry in Munich and its leader, Ernst Ruedin. Indeed, even after his exile, Kallmann continued to see Ruedin as a skilled colleague whose publications would be a great addition to the research literature being published in the United States of America, as this passage from a personal letter to Franz Boas at Columbia reveals:

> It can be seen from numerous examples that researchers in totalitarian countries are not free from political pressure with regard to their choice of research subjects, scientific concepts and publications. This is particularly well illustrated in the areas of human genetics and demographic studies. [...] Even the great authority of German psychiatric genetics, Professor Ernst Ruedin, head of one of the world's largest, oldest and best financed research centers now appears [...] to be hindered to finish his long-term, highly sponsored and extensive studies on the heredity of genius. [...] If it is really the case that the scientific results of his research have no chance of getting past the censorship of today's political leaders [of Nazi Germany], I am convinced that every publishing house, magazine and scientific institute of a democratic country with freedom to research such as America would be pleased to support Dr. Ruedin in publishing such unwanted research results. (Kallmann 1939)[14]

If they seemed "strange bedfellows," it should not entirely surprise us that Kallmann felt some personal appreciation toward his former director. From Ruedin, he received help in leaving Germany and finding a job in the United States of America, and Ruedin's former collaborator, Theodor Lange, brought a collection of data material from Munich to New York City (see Fig. 5). In return, Ruedin received a de-Nazification certificate after 1945 from Kallmann who was already further cooperating again with the eminent

---

[14]Franz Josef Kallmann, Letter to Franz Boas at Columbia University (February 2, 1939); Boas Collection of the Archives of the Library of Congress, Washington, D. C., United States (LOC, Franz Boas Collection, 1939, Microfilm, Fond No. MSS60202).

TABLE 4. DISTRIBUTION OF MARRIED PERSONS (OVER AGE 45) WITH AND WITHOUT CHILDREN IN NORMAL (240) AND PSYCHOTIC (300) TWIN INDEX SIBSHIPS

| TYPE OF TWIN INDEX CASE | WITHOUT CHILDREN | | | | WITH CHILDREN | | | |
| | Twin Subjects | | Sibs | | Twin Subjects | | Sibs | |
	PS	O	PS	O	PS	O	PS	O
Schizophrenic...........	26	27	7	87	104	47	22	275
Manic-Depressive..............	8	1	4	9	18	11	7	53
Senescent (Over Age 60).........		46		45		162		211

PS = With Psychosis   O = Without Psychosis.

TABLE 5. MARITAL REPRODUCTIVITY IN NORMAL (240) AND PSYCHOTIC (300) TWIN FAMILY UNITS

| TYPE OF TWIN INDEX CASE | NUMBER OF CHILDREN PER FERTILE MARRIED PERSON OVER AGE 45 | | | | NUMBER OF CHILDREN PER MARRIED PERSON OVER AGE 45 | | | |
| | Twin Subjects | | Sibs | | Twin Subjects | | Sibs | |
	PS	O	PS	O	PS	O	PS	O
Schizophrenic..............	2.6	2.8	2.1*	3.0*	2.4	1.8	1.2*	2.3*
Manic-Depressive...........	2.1	2.6	2.6	3.0	1.6	2.2	2.0	2.5
Senescent (Over Age 60)......		3.0		3.2		2.4		2.6

PS = With psychosis   O = Without psychosis
* Statistically significant

Figure 5. Franz Kallmann's statistical depiction of the distribution of mental illness (the two major types: schizophrenic and manic-depressive disorders), as he had already worked out in 1941, based on his new methodology (as in Kallmann, 1938b; Kallmann & Bondy 1952).

psychiatrist and eugenicist Theobald Lang (1898–1957), formerly a scientific member of the German Research Institute for Psychiatry and, later, the Kaiser Wilhelm Institute for Racial Anthropology in Berlin. All of this strikingly shows how the international networks in eugenics, human genetics, and biological psychiatry continued on — nearly unchanged — after the end of the Second World War (Hammerstein, 2000, pp. 214–219).

As Gerald Grob has demonstrated in many of his well-researched publications, the predominantly "biophobic attitude" among North American clinical psychiatrists was to a large extent a result of the immense influence of a specific group of émigrés: The psycho-analysts probably shaped the fields of psychiatry, mental health, and psychology more than any other group affected by forced migration. Similar to Kallmann's development, the prevailing trend of reductionism in psychiatric and neurological research at the National Institute of Mental Health proved to be highly influential during the second part of the twentieth century. As these two fields were strongly supported through its extramural program and held strong ties with the clinical research branch, frictions between the various disciplines were inevitable as they competed to draw the research orientation and support of the National Institute of Mental Health (Farreras, Hannahway, & Harden, 2004, pp. 312–315). Similar to Kallmann's own development, the prevailing trend of reductionism in psychiatric and neurological research at the National Institute of Mental Health proved to be highly influential during the second part of the twentieth century.

Looking at the example of early brain research activities supported by the intramural and extramural funding programs of the National Institutes of Health, the biographies of

Kallmann and others tell us much about the actual production of medical and neuroscientific knowledge as a distinctive mirror. We see global history represented in very specific local milieus. As a general trend, the *Machtergreifung* of the Nazis destroyed the early careers and ambitions that many researchers had cultivated up to the end of the Weimar period. All of the émigré neuroscientists in the 1930s and 1940s came into preexisting clinical and research settings in North America, bringing their own specific interplay of conceptual, personal, and organizational relationships, originating from very different research environments (Magoun, 2002, pp. 151–153). However, it is problematic to overstate the differences and to downplay the active, international collaboration occurring in biological psychiatry in the interwar and postwar periods. Certainly, Kallmann's views on the problem of schizophrenia and other severe mental illnesses could have been, and were, voiced on both sides of the Atlantic:

> Schizophrenic taints deteriorate the affected family stocks so consistently that even the best social conditions and the most favorable environment are unable to produce biologically satisfactory individuals and are so widespread that schizophrenic patients make up, in America as elsewhere, the majority of the resident population in mental hospitals [...]. From a eugenic point of view, it is particularly disastrous that these patients not only continue to crowd mental hospitals all over the world, but also afford, to society as a whole, an unceasing source of maladjusted cranks, asocial eccentrics and the lowest types of criminal offenders. Even the faithful believer in the predominance of individual liberty will admit that mankind would be much happier without those numerous adventurers, fanatics and pseudo-saviors of the world who are found again and again to come from the schizophrenic genotype. (Kallmann, 1938b, p. 110)

Acknowledgments

We are grateful for support from the Mackie Family Collection in the History of Neuroscience, the Hotchkiss Brain Institute, the O'Brien Institute for Public Health (all: Calgary, Canada), the Library of Congress (Washington, DC), and the Richardson History of Psychiatry Research Seminar, Cornell University (New York City). We also wish to include Dr. Alan N. Schechter, National Institutes of Health (Bethesda, MD) for his kind assistance and sharing of information during the research process for this article.

Funding

We acknowledge the support of the Ethics Office of the Canadian Institutes of Health Research as well as an Open Operating Grant (no/EOG-123690) from CIHR.

References

Aly G (1994): Medicine against the useless. In: Aly G, Chroust P, Pross C, eds., *Cleansing the Fatherland: Nazi Medicine and Racial Hygiene*, Cooper B, trans. Baltimore, London, The Johns Hopkins University Press, pp. 22–98.

Ash M, Soellner A, eds. (1996): *Forced Migration and Scientific Change: Émigré German–speaking Scientists after 1933*. Cambridge, Cambridge University Press.

Benbassat CA (2016): Kallmann Syndrome: Eugenics and the man behind the eponym. *Rambam Maimonides Medical Journal* 7. Advance online publication. doi: 10.5041/RMMJ.10242

Born G (2011): Refugee scientists in a new environment. In: Marks S, Weindling P, Wintour L, eds., *In Defence of Learning: The Plight, Persecution, and Placement of Academic Refugees, 1933–1980s*. Oxford, Oxford University Press, pp. 77–86.

Cornwell J (2003): *Hitler's Scientists: Science, War, and the Devil's Pact*. New York, Viking Press.

Cottebrune A (2009): Franz Josef Kallmann (1897–1965) und der Transfer psychiatrisch-genetischer Wissenschaftskonzepte vom NS-Deutschland in die USA. *Medizinhistorisches Journal* 44: 296–324.

Davie MR, Koenig S (1949): Adjustment of refugees to American life. *Annals of the American Academy of Political and Social Science* 262: 159–165.

Dodé C, Hardelin JP (2010): Clinical genetics of Kallmann syndrome. *Annals of Endocrinology* 71: 149–157.

Duckett S, Stern J (1999): Origins of the Creutzfeldt and Jakob Concept. *Journal of the History of the Neurosciences* 8: 21–34.

Engstrom E (2003): *Clinical Psychiatry in Imperial Germany: A History of Psychiatric Practice*. New York, Cornell University Press.

Erlenmayer-Kimling L, Falek A, Jarvik LF, Rainer JD, Sank D (1965): Franz Joseph Kallmann, 1897–1965. *Eugenics Quarterly* 12: 123.

Essen-Moeller E (1941): *Psychiatrische Untersuchungen an einer Serie von Zwillingen*. Munksgaard, Acta Psychiatrica et Neurologica, Supplemental Volume 23.

Farreras IG, Hannaway C, Harden, VA, eds. (2004): *Mind, Brain, Body, and Behavior: Foundations of Neuroscience and Behavioral: Research at the National Institutes of Health*. Amsterdam, Rodopi.

Gershon ES (1981): The historical context of Franz Kallmann and psychiatric genetics. *Archiv fuer Psychiatrie und Nervenkrankheiten* 229: 273–276.

Griesinger W (1867): *Mental Pathology and Therapeutics* (Germ. ed. 1845). London, England, New Sydenham Society.

Grob GN (1983): *Mental Illness and American Society: 1875–1940*. Princeton, Princeton University Press.

Grob GN (2000): Mental health policy in late twentieth century America. In: Menninger, RW, Nemiah, JC, eds., *American Psychiatry after World War II (1944–1994)*. Washington, DC, American Psychiatric Press, pp. 232–258.

Hammerstein N (2000): *Die Deutsche Forschungsgemeinschaft in der Zeit der Weimarer Republik und im Dritten Reich: Wissenschaftspolitik in Republik und Diktatur*. Munich, C. H. Beck.

Holdorff B (2016): Emigrated neuroscientists from Berlin to North America. *Journal of the History of the Neurosciences* 25: 227–252.

Joseph J (2006): *The Missing Gene: Psychiatry, Heredity, and the Fruitless Search for Genes*. New York, Algora Publishing.

Joseph J, Wetzel NA (2013): Ernst Ruedin: Hitler's racial hygiene mastermind. *Journal of the History of Biology* 46: 1–30.

Kallmann FJ (1921): *Zufaellige Stichverletzungen als Todesursache*. MD thesis, Breslau, Friedrich Wilhelms University.

Kallmann FJ (1938a): *The Genetics of Schizophrenia: A Study of Heredity and Reproduction of the Families of 1,087 Schizophrenics*. New York, JJ Augustin.

Kallmann FJ (1938b): Heredity, reproduction and eugenic procedure in the field of schizophrenia. *Eugenical News* 23: 105–113.

Kallmann FJ (1939): Informal discussion of sources of mental disease: Amelioration and prevention. In Mouton FR, ed., *Mental Health: Publication of the American Association for the Advancement of Science*. New York, Science Press, pp. 48–62.

Kallmann FJ (1945): Heredity and eugenics. *American Journal of Psychiatry* 102: 522–524.

Kallmann FJ (1950): The genetics of psychoses: An analysis of 1,232 twin index families. *American Journal of Human Genetics* 4: 385–390.

Kallmann FJ (1952): Human genetics as a science, a profession, and as a social-minded trend of orientation. *American Journal of Human Genetics* 4: 237–245.

Kallmann FJ (1956): The genetics of human behavior. *American Journal of Psychiatry* 113: 496–501.

Kallmann FJ (1963): That rare specimen — A psychiatrist concerned with genetics (originally unpublished). *Behavioral Sciences* 11: 292 (excerpt).

Kallmann FJ, Bondy E (1952): Applicability of the twin study method in the analysis of variations in mate selection and marital adjustment. *American Journal of Human Genetics* 4: 209–222.

Kallmann FJ, Schoenfeld WA, Barrera SE (1943–1944): The genetic aspects of primary eunuchoidism. *American Journal of Mental Deficiencies* 48: 203–236.

Kandel ER (1998): A new intellectual framework for psychiatry. *American Journal of Psychiatry* 155: 257–269.

Kaplan HI, Sadock BJ (1995): *Comprehensive Textbook of Psychiatry VI*. New York, Williams & Wilkins, Volume 1.

Kater M (1992): Unresolved questions of German medicine and medical history in the past and present. *Central European History* 25: 407–423.

Kety S (1954): *Annual Reports of the National Institutes of Mental Health*. Bethesda, MD, National Institutes of Health.

Koehler PJ, Stahnisch FW (2014): Three twentieth-century multiauthored neurological handbooks — A historical analysis and bibliometric comparison. *Journal of the History of the Neurosciences* 23: 1–30.

Kroener HP (1998): *Von der Rassenhygiene zur Humangenetik: Das Kaiser-Wilhelm-Institut fuer Anthropologie, menschliche Erblehre und Eugenik nach dem Kriege*. Stuttgart, Gustav Fischer.

Magoun HW (2002): *American Neuroscience in the Twentieth Century: Confluence of the Neural, Behavioral, and Communicative Streams*, Edited and annotated by LH Marshall. Lisse, A. A. Balkema Publishers.

Marcuse H, Kallmann FJ (1929): Zur Sulfosinbehandlung der Paralyse und Schizophrenie. *Nervenarzt* 2: 149–153.

Medawar J, Pyke D (2001): *Hitler's Gift: The True Story of the Scientists Expelled by the Nazi Regime*. New York, Arkade Publishing.

Mehler B (1988): *A History of the American Eugenics Society, 1921–1940*. PhD thesis, Urbana, University of Illinois.

Mildenberger F (2002): Auf der Spur des "Scientific Pursuit" Franz Josef Kallmann (1897–1965) und die rassenhygienische Forschung. *Medizinhistorisches Journal* 37: 183–200.

Panse F (1966): Zur Erinnerung an Franz Kallmann 1897–1965. *Archiv fuer Psychiatrie und Zeitschrift fuer die gesamte Neurologie* 208: I–IV.

Pearle KM (1984): Aerzteemigration nach 1933 in die USA: Der Fall New York. *Medizinhistorisches Journal* 19: 112–137.

Peters UH (1996): Emigration deutscher Psychiater nach England (Teil 1). *Fortschritte der Neurologie und Psychiatrie* 64: 161–167.

Pickenhain L (2002): Die Neurowissenschaft–ein interdisziplinaeres und integratives Wissensgebiet. *Schriftenreihe der Deutschen Gesellschaft fuer Geschichte der Nervenheilkunde* 8: 241–246.

Rainer JD (1966): The contributions of Franz Josef Kallmann to the genetics of schizophrenia. *Behavioral Sciences* 11: 413.

Rainer JD (1972): Perspectives on the genetics of schizophrenia: A re-evaluation of Kallmann's contribution — Its influence and current relevance. *Psychiatric Quarterly* 46: 356–362.

Rheinberger HJ (2005): Reassessing the historical epistemology of Georges Canguilhem. In: Gutting G, ed., *Continental Philosophy of Science*. Maldan, MA, Blackwell Publishing, pp. 187–197.

Ritter J, Roelcke V (2005): Psychiatric genetics in Munich and Basel between 1925 and 1945: Programs – Practices – Cooperative Arrangements. *Osiris* 20: 263–288.

Roelcke V (2006): Funding the scientific foundations of race policies: Ernst Ruedin and the impact of career resources on psychiatric genetics, ca. 1910–1945. In: Eckart WU, ed., *Man, Medicine, and the State: The Human Body as an Object of Government Sponsored Medical Research in the 20th Century*. Stuttgart, Franz Steiner, pp. 73–87.

Roelcke V (2007): Die Etablierung der psychiatrischen Genetik in Deutschland, Grossbritannien und den USA, ca. 1910–1960: Zur untrennbaren Geschichte von Eugenik und Humangenetik. *Acta Historica Leopoldina* 48: 173–190.

Rose N, Abi-Rached JM (2013): *Neuro — The New Brain Sciences and the Sciences of the Mind*. Princeton, Oxford, Princeton University Press.

Shorter E (2005): *A Historical Dictionary of Psychiatry*. Oxford, Oxford University Press.

Slater E (1965): Obituary notices: F. J. Kallmann, M.D. *British Medical Journal* 1: 1440.

Slater E (1968): A review of earlier evidence on genetic factors in schizophrenia. In: Rosenthal D, Kety S, eds., *The Transmission of Schizophrenia*. New York, Pergamon Press, pp. 15–26.

Stahnisch FW (2009): Transforming the lab: Technological and societal concerns in the pursuit of de- and regeneration in the German morphological neurosciences, 1910–1930. *Medicine Studies: An International Journal for History, Philosophy, and Ethics of Medicine & Allied Sciences* 1: 41–54.

Stahnisch FW (2010): German-speaking émigré neuroscientists in North America after 1933: Critical reflections on emigration-induced scientific change. *Oesterreichische Zeitschrift fuer Geschichtswissenschaften (Vienna)* 21: 36–68.

Stahnisch FW (2014): The early eugenics movement and emerging professional psychiatry: Conceptual transfers and personal relationships between Germany and North America, 1880s to 1930s. *Canadian Bulletin of Medical History* 31: 17–40.

Stahnisch FW (2016a): Die Neurowissenschaften in Strassburg zwischen 1872 und 1945: Forschungsaktivitaeten zwischen politischen und kulturellen Zaesuren. *Sudhoffs Archiv. Zeitschrift fuer Wissenschaftsgeschichte* 101: 1–33 (in print).

Stahnisch FW (2016b): From "nerve fiber regeneration" to "functional changes" in the human brain — On the paradigm-shifting work of the experimental physiologist Albrecht Bethe (1872–1954) in Frankfurt am Main. *Frontiers in Systems Neuroscience* 10: 1–16.

Stahnisch FW (2016c): Learning soft skills the hard way: Historiographical considerations on the cultural adjustment process of German-speaking émigré neuroscientists in Canada, 1933 to 1963. *Journal of the History of the Neurosciences* 25: 299–319.

Torrey EF, Yolken RH (1966): Obituary — Franz Joseph Kallmann, 1897–1965. *The American Journal of Psychiatry* 123: 105–106.

Weber MM (1993): *Ernst Ruedin: Eine kritische Biographie*. Berlin, Springer.

Weber MM (2000): Psychiatric research and science policy in Germany: The history of the Deutsche Forschungsanstalt fuer Psychiatrie (German Institute for Psychiatric Research) in Munich from 1917 to 1945. *History of Psychiatry* 11: 235–258.

Weindling PJ (1989): *Health, Race and German Politics between National Unification and Nazism, 1870–1945*. Cambridge, Cambridge University Press.

Weindling P, von Villiez A, Loewenau A, Faron N (2016): The victims of unethical human experiments and coerced research under national socialism. *Endeavour* 40: 1–6.

Zalashik R (2012): *Das unselige Erbe: Die Geschichte der Psychiatrie in Palaestina und Israel*, Ajchenrand D, trans. Frankfurt am Main, Campus Verlag.

Émigré scientists and the global turn in the history of science: A commentary on the volume "Forced Migration in the History of 20th-Century Neuroscience and Psychiatry"

Delia Gavrus

Department of History, University of Winnipeg, Winnipeg, Manitoba, Canada

The articles in this special issue of the *Journal of the History of the Neurosciences* explore the historical realities of the forced migration of physicians and scientists who worked in the middle decades of the twentieth century in the broad area of the mind and brain sciences — the disciplines that will eventually, in the 1970s, be known as the neurosciences. Starting in the early 1930s with the Nazis' rise to power, an increasingly dangerous political environment that culminated in the horrific persecution (personal, professional, financial), the incarceration, and the murder of Jewish scientists led many members of the community to flee Germany for the United States, Canada, the United Kingdom, France, Scandinavia, Turkey, and other countries. They were joined by many other Jewish people, including scholars from other fields of study, intellectuals, and academics, as well as by a much smaller percentage of German and Austrian scientists who, while not Jewish themselves, faced persecution for opposing Nazism. The exodus of these men and women, the tortuous road to safety, and to a regained semblance of professional normality left a crucial mark on the history of their disciplines and more generally on postwar culture (Marks, Weindling, & Wintour, 2011). The authors of the articles in this special issue offer solid empirical investigations that illuminate the historical process as it pertains to a number of scientists working in the area of the brain, mind sciences, and medicine. The authors also lay out a vision for the study of émigré scientists more generally, a vision that resonates with recent historiographical approaches in the history of science that emphasize global communities and the circulation of knowledge.

Over the past few decades, the cross-border movement of science and its practitioners has become a rich area of research for historians and other scholars in the humanities. A historiographical focus on the circulation of knowledge has allowed historians to complicate simplistic ideas of the discovery and spread of knowledge, practices, and technologies, as well as to identify the factors that contributed to the success or failure of such circulation in particular situations (Raj, 2007; Lightman, McOuat, & Stewart, 2013; Cook & Walker, 2013). This scholarship has contributed to a recent "global turn" in the history of science (Sivasundaram, 2010; McCook, 2013; Fan, 2012; Monnais & Cook, 2012), an approach that decentralizes particular geographic locations as centers of knowledge production and instead emphasizes communication, exchange, interaction, and movement that transcends national boundaries. "Circulation" and "movement" are not meant to imply just free circulation or voluntary movement. Similarly, change resulting from scientists' emigration cannot be characterized simply in terms of gains and losses, because change is not subject to such simple arithmetic. As historians Mitchell Ash and Alfons Soellner have noted in the context of the forced migration of German-speaking scholars, "To inquire only about losses and gains in this sense presupposes a static view of science and of culture, as though the émigrés brought with them finished bits of knowledge, which they then inserted like building-stones into already established cultural constructs elsewhere" (1996, p. 4).

The articles of this special issue make this point abundantly clear. Bernd Holdorff examines a number of German-trained scientists and medical students from the Berlin area, showing how difficult it was for the older professionals in particular to find jobs and to adapt to their new environment, even as some of them — Fritz Heinrich Lewy for instance — made lasting contributions to science in his new country. Frank W. Stahnisch shows that those neurologists and psychiatrists who were forced to migrate to Canada did not simply pick up in their professional lives where they had left off in their German-speaking countries. Often, they had to change their work to fit the research agendas or the clinical settings that were viable in Canada. This was, for instance, the case with Karl Stern, who had been trained as a basic science researcher and ended up as a clinician and medical educator in Montreal. Furthermore, as Stahnisch shows, homesickness, the yearning for the home country, was a constant theme in the lives of the displaced men and women.

In her article, Aleksandra Loewenau examines the ways in which German-speaking neurologists, psychiatrists, neuropathologists, and neurosurgeons were helped by relief organizations in Britain. In particular, the Society for the Protection of Sciences and Learning and the Rockefeller Foundation were instrumental in finding academic and medical positions for some of the refugee doctors and scientists. Many doctors, however, were turned down by the British medical establishment. Loewenau also shows that younger men were more likely to have their application processed faster, while older scientists faced a longer waiting period and had more difficulty finding a position. Discrepancies in the ability to attain a position are also evident with respect to the refugees' expertise. Thus, psychiatrists were more in demand than other medical specialists, partly due to their research expertise and partly due to the fact that the discipline was seen to be lagging behind in Britain.

In their article, Lawrence A. Zeidman, Anna von Villiez, Jan-Patrick Stellmann, and Hendrik van den Bussche focus on five scientists of Jewish descent who were forced to abandon their lives in Hamburg and to flee abroad. In many cases, a sort of "double emigration" ensued, until the men reached a country in which they could settle. Some of these scientists had to endure not just the crushing loss of their professional positions, their medical licenses, and their material assets but they were also subjected to deportation and internment in concentration camps. Even when, after being itinerant for a while, they settled and obtained work, it took them years to attain positions on par to the ones they had left behind, if they ever attained such positions at all. As Zeidman, von Villiez, Stellmann, and van den Bussche succinctly put it, "the brain drain did not equal a 'brain gain.'"

Even in countries where high-paid university positions were offered to Jewish academics forced to leave their German-speaking countries, these individuals still had to grapple with difficult issues of identity and the process of having left behind family, friends, working relationships, and material assets, as Gül Russell shows in her article on émigré scientists who went to Turkey. The experimental psychologist Wilhelm Peters, who after a brief stay in Britain obtained a position at Istanbul University, struggled with the new language and with a university environment that was much less rich than the one he had left behind. Despite many challenges, including xenophobic sentiments from some nationalist colleagues, Peters was eventually successful in establishing an Institute of Experimental Psychology. Russell illustrates how, due to the political climate in Turkey, Jewish émigrés such as Peters had to contend with the presence of other academics who were German spies and Nazi informers and who made the already uncomfortable environment of a foreign country even more unpleasant for émigrés and for other Turkish scholars. In the latter category, the psychologist Muzafer Sherif denounced fascist ideology and as a communist he was imprisoned in Turkey and had to move to the United States, becoming himself a displaced scholar.

The story of another displaced scholar sheds light on the relationship between forced migration and knowledge circulation. The career of geneticist Franz Josef Kallmann exemplifies the disturbing connection between eugenic ideology in Nazi Germany and in the United States, as Stephen Pow and Frank W. Stahnisch show in their article. Forced to emigrate to the United States because his Jewish ancestry was putting him at risk in Nazi Germany, Kallmann brought with him an interest and expertise in the study of genetics and mental illness. Despite the fact that in the U.S. the academic milieu favored an environmentalist and psychoanalytic approach to mental health, Kallmann did well for himself professionally, assuming important leadership roles and eventually being celebrated by some as a pioneering figure in biological psychiatry. His favored research methodology — twin studies, through which he attempted to tease out the role of heredity — were widely adopted by behavioral geneticists in the second half of the 20th century, as a focus on biology displaced the previously popular psychoanalytic framework. But, as Pow and Stahnisch show, Kallmann maintained more than just a biological orientation in his American career; he also retained his support of eugenic ideas and policies — and, shockingly, he did so without seeming to incur professional penalties for his views on sterilization programs, or for his continuing ties with Nazi psychiatric researchers and policy makers like Ernst Ruedin, who played an active role in Nazi atrocities. Kallmann's example shows, as Pow and Stahnisch argue, the inescapable historical ties between some early research in the field of psychiatric genetics and eugenics ideology and policies on both sides of the Atlantic. The forced migration of researchers contributed to the circulation of such ideas as well.

Collectively, the articles in this volume show how the history of the mind and brain sciences and the history of neuroscience in the twentieth century can contribute a great deal to historiographical issues that currently interest historians of science, and especially to the global turn and the emphasis on the circulation of knowledge. In this context, there are several important overarching themes that emerge from these articles.

First, the issue of national styles of doing and thinking about the sciences is echoed by several authors, and an analysis of the ways in which these national styles clash and inform each other can form the basis of a global approach to the study of transnational scientific communities. Historians of science have long identified the differences in method, organization, funding, values, and interests that determine the scope and the performance of science in various national contexts (see, for instance, Harwood, 1993). As some of the articles in this volume demonstrate, this was also the case with the sciences of the nervous system. Disciplinary boundaries (such as those between neurology and neuropsychiatry) and research commitments (such as holistic versus reductionist approaches to brain research) were starkly distinctive in different geographical regions, and the former education and professional experience of the émigré scientists sometimes carried a serious liability when it came to finding a position in the new country. To complicate matters, these émigrés were arriving, in the 1930s and 1940s, in the middle of a vigorous debate among North American neurologists, psychiatrists, and neurosurgeons about the boundaries and the scope of these related medical specialties (Gavrus, 2011). All these factors raise fascinating questions about the global and international aspects of these science and research fields. How can historians best describe the heterogeneous transnational community of the mind and brain sciences during and after World War II, especially in light of the émigrés' experiences? To what extent did the émigré scientists feel that they were part of a global scientific community in their particular disciplines? How were their professional networks disrupted or enhanced by the forced migration? Is the case of neuroscience similar to or different from that of molecular biology, which, as historian Pnina Abir-Am has shown, "has primarily constituted itself in an international space" (1993, p. 153) in exactly the same time period and due, in no small measure, to the movement of scientists across national borders?

Secondly, the contributions to this special issue highlight some of the factors that play a powerful role in shaping postmigration life, and, in so doing, the articles speak to a much larger literature that delves into the process of adaptation and reverse migration that émigrés in different times and situations have experienced. In the case of the mind and brain sciences and medicine, the émigrés' different approaches to scientific and medical practice may have very well led to what Stahnisch and Russell call "the emergence of interdisciplinarity" while, as Holdorff suggests, the best chances for a successful transition belonged to those who were young students at the time of their refuge. Age is thus one of the powerful factors that can potentially shape adaptation. Furthermore, the frequent transitions that the older men experienced — from job to job, from country to country, from freedom to imprisonment even once they were outside Germany — took an incredible toll on their emotional well-being. And, as other historians have shown, discrimination was a common fact of life in the émigrés' new countries. Once the Jewish scientists and scholars arrived in the United States, they faced a pervasive culture of anti-Semitism that affected not only their ordinary daily interactions but also the academic and research settings in which they were attempting to work. The reluctance of the universities to hire Jewish academics began to decline only slowly, partly as the result of some philanthropic organizations' policy of "exerting pressure gently and appealing to the self-interests of American institutions of higher education" (Lamberti, 2006, p. 192).

It is instructive to compare this reality with that of a different set of immigrants who were welcomed into Canada starting with the 1950s: foreign-trained doctors. These professionals were recruited in order to make up for the low number of Canadian-trained doctors, and their histories of migration were completely different, as historians David Wright and Sasha Mullally demonstrate. These doctors exchanged much less advantageous professional positions, usually in the United Kingdom, for better positions and professional freedom, since the medical profession in Canada was more egalitarian than its hierarchical British counterpart (Wright, Mullally, & Cordukes,

2010; Mullally & Wright, 2008).[1] As Zeidman, von Villiez, Stellmann, and van den Bussche note in this special issue "'emigration' is a voluntary move from one country to another, not being disenfranchised to the point where leaving, if possible, is the only viable option." It may be instructive then to look at these two literatures — on the voluntary and the involuntary migration of physicians and scientists in the middle of the twentieth century — in order to fully understand the unique details of each case and in order to see how factors such as age or career stage could have profoundly different effects in these different contexts. A similarly productive rapprochement can be sought with the literature on other twentieth-century forms of exile, such as the forced exodus (and, in some cases, the subsequent repatriation) of writers from the communist block — a literature that emphasizes the legal difficulties of both leaving and settling, and which offers a conceptual exploration of the notions of home, homelessness, and homesickness (Neubauer & Toeroek, 2009).

Thus, by focusing on migration, immigration, and exile, historians of neuroscience can participate in a rich conversation with the broader scholarly community and can contribute especially to the recent global turn in the history of science. In turn, this historiographic focus will complicate the brain-drain/gain dichotomy, will raise questions about transnational professional identity, will illuminate networks of knowledge-sharing and will make visible the interplay between the local and the global in the production of science.

Lastly, a general theme that emerges from the articles in this special issue is that of remembrance. It is clear that, after the war, many of the German-speaking scientists who either replaced their displaced Jewish colleagues or who were quiet in the face of such outrageous injustice did not make amends for their behavior or attempt to "repair an open wound," as Zeidman, von Villiez, Stellmann, and van den Bussche put it. Keeping this history alive through historical research and through special-focus issues such as this one perhaps offers a way to stay engaged in that necessary process of healing.

Acknowledgments

The author would like to thank Daniel Stone, Frank Stahnisch, and the anonymous reviewers for their very helpful comments and suggestions.

References

Abir-Am P (1993): From multidisciplinary collaboration to transnational objectivity: International space as constitutive of molecular biology, 1930–1970. In: Crawford ET, Shinn T, Soerlin S, eds., *Denationalizing Science: The Contexts of International Scientific Practice*. Dordrecht, Kluwer Academic Publishers, pp. 153–186.

Ash MG, Soellner A, eds. (1996): *Forced Migration and Scientific Change: Emigre German-Speaking Scientists and Scholars after 1933*. Cambridge, Cambridge University Press.

Cook HJ, Walker TD (2013): Circulation of medicine in the early modern Atlantic world. *Social History of Medicine* 26(3): 337–351.

Fan F (2012): The global turn in the history of science. *East Asian Science, Technology and Society: An International Journal* 6(2): 249–258.

---

[1] As the authors show, South Asian physicians who felt discriminated against in the UK also opted for Canada in large numbers, though some provinces, like Ontario, still discriminated against them.

Gavrus D (2011): Men of dreams and men of action: Neurologists, neurosurgeons, and the performance of professional identity, 1920–1950. *Bulletin of the History of Medicine* 85(1): 57–92.

Harwood J (1993): *Styles of Scientific Thought: The German Genetics Community, 1900–1933, Science and Its Conceptual Foundations.* Chicago, University of Chicago Press.

Lamberti M (2006): The reception of refugee scholars from Nazi Germany in America: Philanthropy and social change in higher education. *Jewish Social Studies* 12(3): 157–192.

Lightman BV, McOuat G, Stewart L, eds. (2013): *The Circulation of Knowledge between Britain, India, and China: The Early-Modern World to the Twentieth Century.* Leiden, Brill, Volume 36.

Marks S, Weindling P, Wintour L, eds. (2011): *In Defence of Learning: The Plight, Persecution, and Placement of Academic Refugees, 1933–1980s.* Oxford, Oxford University Press, Volume 169.

McCook S (2013): Focus: Global Currents in national histories of science: The "Global Turn" and the history of science in Latin America. *Isis* 104(4): 773–776.

Monnais L, Cook HJ (2012): *Global Movements, Local Concerns: Medicine and Health in Southeast Asia.* Singapore, NUS Press.

Mullally S, Wright D (2008): La grande séduction?: The immigration of foreign-trained physicians to Canada, C. 1954–76. *Journal of Canadian Studies/Revue d'études canadiennes* 41(3): 67–89.

Neubauer J, Török BZ, eds. (2009): *The Exile and Return of Writers from East-Central Europe: A Compendium.* Berlin, Walter de Gruyter.

Raj K (2007): *Relocating Modern Science: Circulation and the Construction of Knowledge in South Asia and Europe, 1650–1900.* New York, Palgrave Macmillan.

Sivasundaram S (2010): Sciences and the global: On methods, questions, and theory. *Isis* 101(1): 146–158.

Wright D, Mullally S, Cordukes MC (2010): "Worse than being married": The exodus of British doctors from the National Health Service to Canada, C. 1955–75. *Journal of the History of Medicine and Allied Sciences* 65(4): 546–575.

Index

Tretiakoff, K.N. 61
Turhan, M. 109, *109*
Turkey 1–2, 7, 145–147; Ankara University 96–97,
112, 118; Atatuerk 95, *96*; Institute of
Experimental Psychology 108, 147; Institute of
Pedagogy 106; Institute of Pedagogy and
Psychology 110, *111*; Istanbul 95–97; Istanbul
University 102–115, *103*; National Socialist
Government 95; Nationalist Socialist Party 95
twenty-first century 96
typology 7

United Kingdom (UK) 2–4, 14, 24–25, 36, 84, 99,
148; Academic Assistance Council (AAC) 12–15,
18, 21, 40–42, 101–102, 145; The Alien's Order 35;
British Medical Association (BMA) 36–37; British
Psychological Association (BPA) 101; Child
Guidance Clinic 99, 108; Home Office 36–39, 98,
101; London 37, 78; London School of Economics
(LSE) 40; Medical Practitioners Union (MPU) 36;
Medical Research Council (MRC) 44, 44n17, 75;
naturalization 38; relief and funding organizations
38, **39**; Royal College of Physicians (RCP) 4
United States of America (USA) 1–7, 48–55, 58–63,
117–119, 123–126, 130–139, 145–148; American
Academy of Neurology (AAN) 4; American
Eugenic Society (AES) 134; American Medical
Association (AMA) 2, 49; American Society of
Human Genetics (ASHG) 134, 137; Boston 48;
California 24–26, 29; Chicago 14–15, 58;
Columbia-Presbyterian Medical Center 135, *136*;
culture 65; Emergency Committee in Aid of
Displaced Foreign Scholars 43, 49, 67, 82; Federal
Bureau of Investigation (FBI) 117; Illinois 14–15,
29; Massachusetts Institute of Technology (MIT)
50–51; National Institute of Health (NIH)
136–138; National Institute of Mental Health
(NIMH) 134, 137, 140; New York 18, 29, 48–49,
63–67, 82, 123–125, 131–132; New York Academy
of Medicine (NYAM) 49; New York State
Psychiatric Institute 133–135; San Francisco 25,
68; Texas 25; Veterans Administration (VA)
Hospital 16, 22
University of Berlin (Germany) 50–52
University of Breslau (Poland) 127

University of Wuerzburg (Germany) 100–103,
107–109

Versailles Treaty (1919) 33–34
Verschuer, O.F. von 132, 135
Veterans Administration (VA) Hospital (USA) 16,
22, 54n4
Vienna (Austria) 40, 110
Villiez, A. von, *et al.* 6, 9–32, 146, 149

Wagenen, W.P. van 60
Wagner-Jauregg, J. 50
Warburg, E. 23
Wartenberg, R. 67–69
Wartenberg's disease 68n17
Weil, R. 7
Weimar Period 76, 102, 105, 141
Weimar Republic 3, 33, 91, 126
Weindling, P. 34, 42
Weizsaecher, R. von 30
Wernicke, C. 54–56, 65
Wertheimer, M. 105, *106*
Weygandt, W. 12, 23
White Russia 34
Wilhelmian policy (Germany, 1897–1914) 104
Wilhelminian Empire 92
Wittkower, E.D. 38, 42, 45
Wood, C. 118, *118*
Woodworth, R.S. 113
World Health Organization (WHO) 89
World War I (1914–1918) 11–14, 18–20, 53, 65, 104,
113, 126–130
World War II (1939–1945) 7, 50–53, 66–69, 87–89,
112–114, 124–125, 138–140
Wright, D. 148
Wundt, W. 100, 103, 105, *105*

xenophobia 49

Yakovlev, P. 22

Zalashik, R. 139
Zeidman, L.A., *et al.* 6, 9–32, 146, 149
Zimmerman, D. 45
Zuckmayer, C. 78

For Product Safety Concerns and Information please contact our EU
representative GPSR@taylorandfrancis.com
Taylor & Francis Verlag GmbH, Kaufingerstraße 24, 80331 München, Germany

www.ingramcontent.com/pod-product-compliance
Ingram Content Group UK Ltd.
Pitfield, Milton Keynes, MK11 3LW, UK
UKHW031043080625
459435UK00013B/546